Healthy Eating Every Day

Ruth Ann Carpenter, MS, RD, LD

Carrie E. Finley, MS

The Cooper Institute

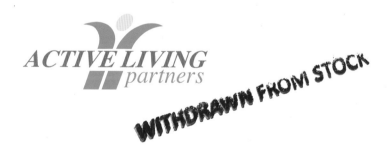

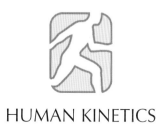

HUMAN KINETICS

Library of Congress Cataloging-in-Publication Data

Carpenter, Ruth Ann, 1958-
  Healthy eating every day / Ruth Ann Carpenter, Carrie E. Finley.
      p. cm.
  Includes bibliographical references and index.
  ISBN 0-7360-5186-4
  1. Nutrition--Popular works. I. Finley, Carrie E., 1975- II. Title.
  RA784.C283 2005
  613.2--dc22

                              2004018478

ISBN: 0-7360-5186-4

The Web addresses cited in this text were current as of September 2004, unless otherwise noted.

Acquisitions Editor: Michele Guerra, MS, CHES; **Developmental Editor:** Christine M. Drews; **Assistant Editor:** Kathleen D. Bernard; **Copyeditor:** Christine M. Drews; **Proofreader:** Kathy Bennett; **Indexer:** Susan Hernandez; **Permission Manager:** Dalene Reeder; **Graphic Designer:** Nancy Rasmus; **Graphic Artist:** Dawn Sills; **Photo Managers:** Kelly Huff, Kareema McLendon; **Cover Designer:** Keith Blomberg; **Photographer (cover):** Kelly Huff; **Photographers (interior):** © Human Kinetics. Photos on pages 1, 7, 61 (bottom right), 73, 105, 133, 156, 157, 175, 177, 188, 192 © Photo Network; ix, 19, 41 (left), 55, 92, 108, 187, 204, 207 © Getty Images; viii, 5, 31, 69 (left) © Bruce Coleman; 57, 69 (right), 127, 171 © Dale Garvey; vii © Jumpfoto; 28 © Sport the Library; 41 (right) © Rhoda Peacher; 61 (top) © Ruth Jensen Orewiler; 67 © Jim and Mary Whitmer; 161 © Jay Weesner; 190 © David Liebman; and 195 © Comstock/Getty images; **Art Manager:** Kelly Hendren; **Illustrators:** Dick Flood, Denise Lowry

Human Kinetics books are available at special discounts for bulk purchase. Special editions or book excerpts can also be created to specification. For details, contact the Special Sales Manager at Human Kinetics.

Printed in Hong Kong   10   9   8   7   6   5   4   3   2   1

Human Kinetics
Web site: www.HumanKinetics.com

United States: Human Kinetics
P.O. Box 5076
Champaign, IL 61825-5076
800-747-4457
e-mail: humank@hkusa.com

Canada: Human Kinetics
475 Devonshire Road Unit 100
Windsor, ON N8Y 2L5
800-465-7301 (in Canada only)
e-mail: orders@hkcanada.com

Europe: Human Kinetics
107 Bradford Road
Stanningley
Leeds LS28 6AT, United Kingdom
+44 (0) 113 255 5665
e-mail: hk@hkeurope.com

Australia: Human Kinetics
57A Price Avenue
Lower Mitcham, South Australia 5062
08 8277 1555
e-mail: liaw@hkaustralia.com

New Zealand: Human Kinetics
Division of Sports Distributors NZ Ltd.
P.O. Box 300 226 Albany
North Shore City
Auckland
0064 9 448 1207
e-mail: blairc@hknewz.com

CONTENTS

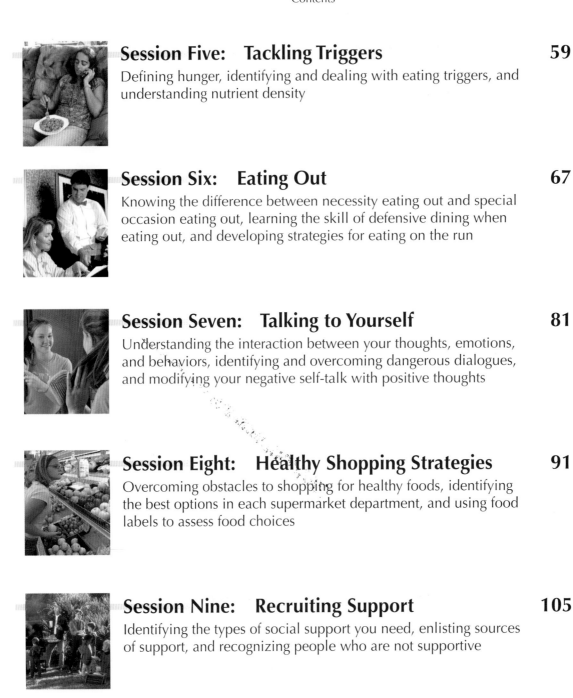
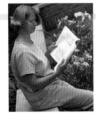

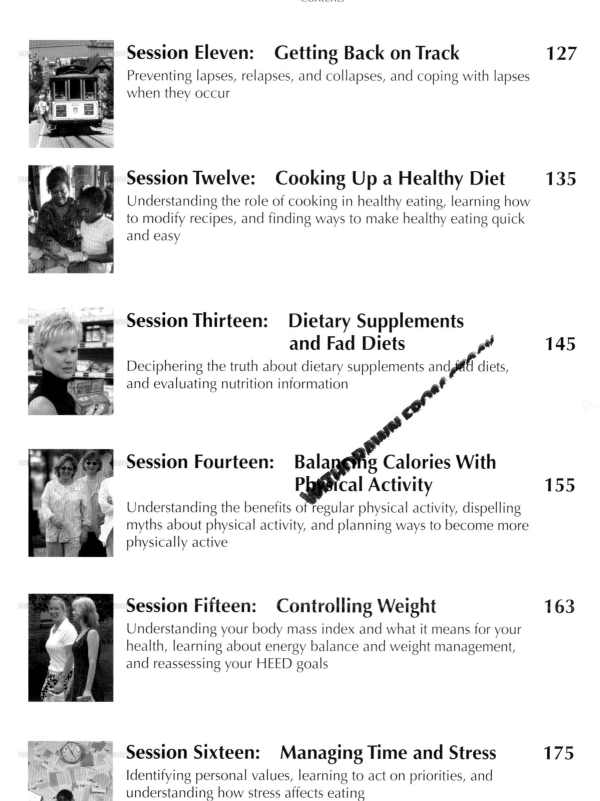

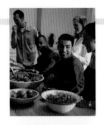
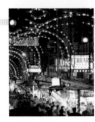
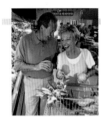
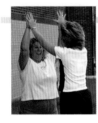

PREFACE

Welcome to *Healthy Eating Every Day!* We're so glad you've picked up this book. By doing so, you've taken a big step to learn more about healthy eating. Because healthy eating can lead to many benefits, including a longer life, more energy, and less chance of serious disease, we know you'll want to stick with us through all 20 sessions. In fact, many people just like you have followed the *Healthy Eating Every Day* plan and have been able to change their eating habits for the better despite years of unhealthy eating. You can do it too!

A Plan to Help You Put Health in Every Bite

Do you need a total diet makeover or just a little tweak here and there? Either way, have we got the plan for you! This book is for you if you . . .

- have ever been told by your doctor that you need to watch what you eat because of problems with high blood pressure, high blood cholesterol, or excess weight;
- want to reduce your risk of developing major lifestyle diseases such as heart disease, cancer, and diabetes as you get older; or
- think that eating better might give you more energy and help you feel better.

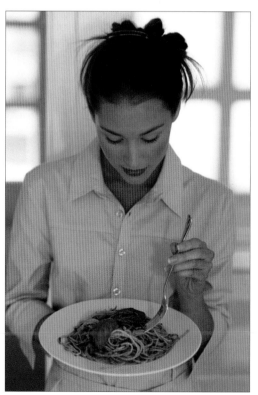

Healthy Eating Every Day can also help most members of your family, because the dietary recommendations provided in this book are appropriate for all generally healthy people above two years of age.

Most books on diet and nutrition tell you a lot about what you shouldn't eat and some about what you should eat. Many require you to make drastic changes in your current eating habits and lifestyle. Some promote practices that are a bit strange or even downright dangerous. Most of all, they promise a quick fix, especially when it comes to weight loss. But the reason so many new diet and nutrition books flood the market each year is that the quick-fix approach doesn't work over time!

This book is different. You will be able to eat every food that you like. We believe that all foods can be part of a healthy diet. You will be able to tailor the recommendations to the specific areas in which *you* need to improve. You'll make gradual changes that over time add up to significant improvements in your nutrient intake and your health. In short, this book will help you put good health in every bite.

How Do We Know It Works?

Healthy Eating Every Day, or HEED as we like to call it, is based on sound research. Each day, new studies point to the importance of diet in the prevention and treatment of common health problems. Much of the research is on the health-protecting effects of specific nutrients such as fat, fiber, cholesterol, vitamin C, and beta-carotene. But mounting evidence shows that eating certain whole foods and food groups—such as fruits, vegetables, whole grains, and low-fat dairy products—independently and in combination, may protect against heart disease, cancer, stroke, obesity, and diabetes. This book was designed to help you focus on eating a balance of foods in a healthy food pattern to improve the quality of your total diet.

We do that by encouraging you to eat a daily diet in line with the Healthy Eating Every Day (HEED) pyramid, a food guide that we have created based on our research and that of other scientists. Most governments' food guides provide good advice for healthy eating, and you will find many similarities among different government food guides and the HEED pyramid. We have simply created a food guide that is more relevant to the goals and approaches of HEED.

In addition to helping you choose a balanced diet, we will help you build and use the lifestyle skills that are necessary to make habit changes permanent. Let's face it: Change is hard. But the latest research shows that learning how to track your food intake, set realistic goals and rewards, cope with triggers for inappropriate eating, seek help from people around you, and apply other behavioral skills increases your chance of making changes last a lifetime. In HEED, we'll take you step-by-step through information and activities that will help you improve your eating habits.

How do we know HEED works? Because it is based on the materials and approaches that were tested in a recent study that we conducted at The Cooper Institute.[1] We recruited 98 generally healthy men and women between the ages of 29 and 71 to participate in a six-month study. After assessing their baseline dietary habits, the participants were randomly assigned to one of three groups.

- One group received a nutrition reference book only. This was called the "usual care group."
- Another group received the nutrition book and the program materials, and attended weekly sessions to review and discuss the program materials. This was called the "weekly meeting group."

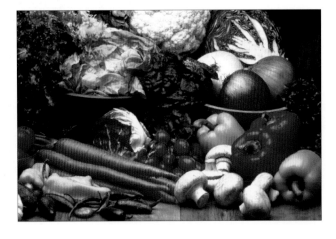

- The third group, the "correspondent group," received the nutrition book and the program materials by mail, and could access a study Web site to participate in weekly chat sessions, post questions, or peruse healthy recipes and restaurant reviews.

The results showed that people who completed the program in the group setting improved their total diet quality more than the other two groups did. But the correspondent group also showed some slight improvements compared to the usual care group. This means that the materials were effective in helping people eat healthier diets, especially people who met regularly with others. We conducted numerous focus group meetings at the end of the study to get feedback from the participants. Overall, they loved the program and made some great suggestions for how we could make it even better! We've incorporated their input into this book.

What About Weight Control?

Most people pick up a book on nutrition because they want to lose weight. If that's you, keep reading. However, we want you to know these things about weight loss:

1. Weight loss and weight control have as much to do with a person's physical activity level as they do with what a person eats. In fact, some scientists believe that exercise is more important than diet in keeping weight off after it is lost!
2. Most weight-loss programs focus on quick weight loss through severe caloric or food restriction. This is unrealistic over the long term and can put you at risk for not getting adequate nutrients.
3. People often don't learn the behavioral skills and strategies that make weight management eating habits stick.

In sessions 14 and 15 we talk about ways to manage your weight by balancing the calories you eat with the calories that you burn through exercise. Other than that, this book doesn't address physical activity in great detail. But we at The Cooper Institute have a lot of experience in helping people move more. In fact, we have translated materials from our very successful research studies into a book and online course called *Active Living Every Day.* The philosophies, approaches, and components of *Active Living Every Day* are very similar to *Healthy Eating Every Day* and are also available from Human Kinetics. For more information, go to www.ActiveLiving.info or call 800-747-4457.

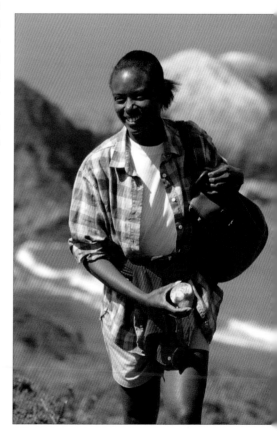

Because HEED doesn't cover physical activity in great detail, you shouldn't expect it to lead to significant weight loss. Still, if you are overweight you will likely lose weight as you learn to manage portion sizes, monitor your caloric intake, and choose low-fat, high-fiber foods. If you are not overweight, improving your diet the HEED way will help you keep the extra weight from piling on in the future. Whether or not you lose weight, you will be eating a healthier diet.

It's More Than a Book

This book is actually one component of a two-part program. In addition to this book, you can also choose to enroll in HEED Online. This Internet-based component will enable you to track your progress, do fun interactive activities, and get additional information, assistance, and links to helpful resources. HEED Online is not a replacement for the book. It works in tandem with the book to provide you with a fun, interesting, and helpful interactive experience to promote healthy eating. To enroll in HEED Online, go to www.ActiveLiving.info or call 800-747-4457.

We want you to be an active participant. After all, healthy eating is a hands-on activity. So learning about healthy eating should be hands-on as well. *Healthy Eating Every Day*—the book and HEED Online—is presented in 20 sessions. We've called them sessions rather than chapters because we want you to experience HEED, not just read about it. Each session contains more than words—you'll find activities, checklists, and thought-provoking questions. To get the most out of HEED, we recommend that you read a session and then take some time to do the activities and apply the information to your life before reading the material in the next session. We have designed HEED so that you can complete one session per week. But you can go faster if you like or take more time if necessary. Keep in mind that change takes time. Giving yourself too much time between sessions may make it too difficult to stay on track. Try to give yourself five to six months to complete HEED.

Each HEED session provides practical information on changing your eating habits. Some of the sessions focus on skills that will help you change your habits. These skills apply to changing almost any habit. Other sessions focus on nutrition skills such as how to eat out, shop, and cook in healthy ways. Although you can use the skills to change any part of your diet, we have selected five strategies that the latest research indicates are most likely to improve health and reduce disease risk. They are also the areas that most people need to change. We've called these five strategies the HEED goals:

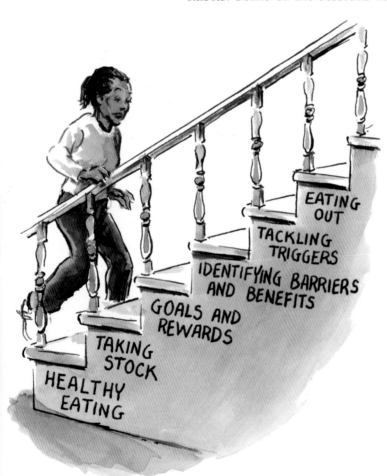

1. Increasing fruits and vegetables
2. Decreasing fats
3. Increasing dairy and dairy alternatives
4. Increasing whole grains
5. Balancing calories

We'll help you target the areas you need to work on and help you set goals that address your particular needs. You'll even have opportunities to change your goals from time to time. For example, you might start with one goal—such as "increasing fruits and vegetables"—and once you have improved in that area, you might switch to focus on another goal.

Early sessions will help you identify exactly what a healthy diet looks like, what's getting in the way of you eating in a healthy manner, and how you can set goals that will lead to lifelong changes. You will then review specific nutrition and behavior change topics such as eating out, confronting eating triggers, getting support, and preventing relapses. Each session is broken down into bite-sized pieces with practical, convenient strategies for making it all work. In addition to the main content that is presented in each session, the following features provide important information throughout the book:

 Nutrition Notes are sections in which you will be asked to write down information.

 Weighty Matters are sidebars that address topics and issues related to weight management.

 Portion Distortion segments provide practical tips for making sure you're using proper portion sizes.

 Science Updates describe in easy-to-understand terms the latest research on the diet and disease connection, healthy eating behavior change strategies, and food science advancements.

 Up Close and Personal stories introduce you to people just like you who are working toward healthy eating every day.

 Did You Know? sections provide information about new items in the stores, fun facts, myth busters, and other interesting food trivia.

Finally, we recognize that healthy eating issues are much the same whether you live in North America, Europe, Australia, New Zealand, or another part of the world. We know that people all over the world might benefit from eating the HEED way. We have made every effort to provide as much inclusive information as possible, and even more can be found in HEED Online.

You want to eat healthier. Good for you! This book is filled with information that can help you achieve your healthy eating goals—from state-of-the-art information on nutrition and behavior change to practical tips and strategies for eating in today's hectic world. We believe that *Healthy Eating Every Day* can help you make healthy eating and good health last a lifetime.

ACKNOWLEDGMENTS

A program of this scale could never be the result of just two people's effort. We are grateful to Mr. Paul E. Dinkel for providing the funding for our Lifestyle Nutrition Study, which proved that the nutrition education approach we have taken in HEED works. We also wish to thank our colleagues Drs. Andrea L. Dunn and Steven N. Blair for their scientific guidance and support of both the Lifestyle Nutrition Study and HEED. Beth Wright, Kherrin Wood, Janet Chandler, Heather Kitzman, Nancy Pierce, Jill Armayor, Marisa Beck, and Doug Gattis provided technical expertise to ensure that the Lifestyle Nutrition Study went smoothly. We learned a tremendous amount from the 98 participants in the Lifestyle Nutrition Study, so we thank them as well.

Many people at The Cooper Institute have put a lot of time and expertise into converting the Lifestyle Nutrition Study materials into the book that you have in your hands and the companion HEED Online. Rachel Coolman and Beth Wright read early drafts and helped us mesh the book content with what appears online. Special thanks to Rachel for her terrific leadership in carrying the learning objectives for each session into the interactive environment of HEED Online (www.ActiveLiving.info). In addition, three very capable interns, Rachelle Fong, Barbara Rodriguez Graf, and Lynn Southard, helped research sources and provided input on many segments.

Regardless of the effort we at The Cooper Institute put into this book, it would still be words on paper without the expert help of many people at Human Kinetics. We thank Rainer Martens and Michele Guerra for sharing in our vision of bringing an evidence-based nutrition education program to consumers. Chris Drews expertly guided us through the reviews and revision process, keeping us on task and always cheering us on with her wonderful upbeat spirit. Jackie Blakley helped us organize the manuscript early on, and Kathleen Bernard made sure no details were left undone. We are also grateful to the many behind-the-scenes players at Human Kinetics who have been involved in the book design and layout, photo acquisition, illustrations, and marketing. It has been a great pleasure working with such talented and dedicated professionals.

Finally, we thank our respective families and our friends for their understanding and support when we spent long hours at nights and on weekends working to make HEED a reality.

ONE

Healthy Eating: A Balancing Act

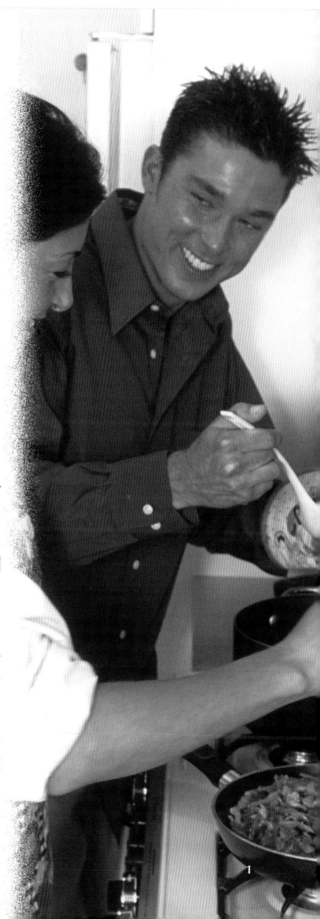

In This Session

- Knowing the importance of dietary balance
- Learning about serving sizes
- Identifying personal improvements in food groups

So you think your eating habits could use some help? You have come to the right place! Regardless of the shape your diet is in today, by the end of *Healthy Eating Every Day* (HEED), you will have learned many skills and strategies to improve your eating habits and to maintain a healthy diet for a lifetime.

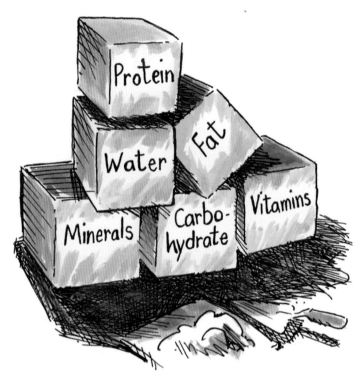

Figure 1.1 Nutrition building blocks.

What exactly is a healthy diet? Many people think it is all about cutting calories or reducing fat to help them lose weight or reduce their risk of heart disease. Indeed, reducing calories and fat has been the focus of many popular "dieting" programs. And it's true that these are goals for most people. But there's much more to healthy eating than reducing calories and fat. For example, you could eat a very low-fat diet but at the same time not get enough milk or calcium-rich foods. This might put you at risk for osteoporosis (weak bones) or other health problems. Likewise, if you cut way back on calories you might not get enough protein, vitamins, or minerals for your body to work well.

Simply put, the foods and beverages we eat and drink are the primary sources of the nutrient building blocks that our bodies need. Our bodies use these nutrients to build tissues, regulate chemical processes, and generate energy to warm and move our bodies. Scientists have long identified these building blocks as protein, different types of carbohydrate, vitamins, minerals, water, and yes, even fat (figure 1.1).

? DID YOU KNOW?

Diet and Disease Connection

Nutrition plays an important role in the prevention of many diseases and health conditions including heart disease, stroke, cancer, obesity, diabetes, and osteoporosis. In fact, some experts estimate that dietary changes could prevent as many as 35% of cancer deaths in many Western countries each year. Think about the difference this could make in your life.

Healthy eating is also essential in treating diseases such as diabetes, heart disease, and cancer. Of course, other factors such as exercising, not smoking, managing stress, and taking medications as prescribed also affect overall health. Whether for prevention or treatment, eating a healthy diet is good medicine.

Recent research has led scientists and health organizations to recommend certain healthy eating patterns. An eating pattern is the usual selection of foods eaten over the course of a day, week, or month. Not all eating patterns are healthy. Skipping breakfast, eating a burger and greasy side dish for lunch, devouring a large steak and potato at dinner, and snacking on sweets would be considered an unhealthy eating pattern. The DASH diet is an example of a healthy eating pattern (see the following Science Update). Many governments' food guidelines offer additional eating pattern recommendations, and we will explore them in more depth later in this session.

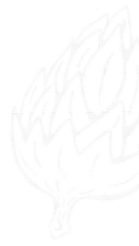 SCIENCE UPDATE

The DASH Diet

Researchers have recently shown that the DASH diet is effective in lowering blood pressure levels and blood cholesterol levels in adults. DASH stands for the Dietary Approaches to Stop Hypertension clinical study. The DASH diet includes limited amounts of lean meats and is high in

- fruits and vegetables (8-10 servings per day),
- low-fat dairy foods (2-3 servings per day),
- whole grains (3 or more servings per day), and
- legumes, nuts, and seeds (4-5 servings per week).

When compared to the control group, which ate a diet with the nutrient intake that is typical for most Americans, those on the DASH diet reduced systolic blood pressure by 5.5 mmHg and diastolic blood pressure by 3.0 mmHg.[2] Blood pressure decreased even more in people who also reduced their sodium intake.[3] Total blood cholesterol level decreased by 13.7 ml/dL.[4] If everyone followed the DASH diet, deaths from heart disease might decrease by 15%. Deaths from stroke might decrease by 27%.[2] The dietary goals of HEED are very similar to those in the DASH diet. ▊

The HEED Approach

The mission of *Healthy Eating Every Day* (HEED) is to help you enjoy better health by bringing your diet in line with the healthy eating patterns promoted by many health and nutrition experts around the world. To assist you, we focus on five dietary changes that most people need to make. We call these the HEED goals:

1. Increasing fruits and vegetables
2. Decreasing fats
3. Increasing dairy products and dairy alternatives
4. Increasing whole grains
5. Balancing calories

We will discuss these more in the next session.

In addition to the five HEED goals, we believe that several attitudes will be important in helping you make lasting changes in your eating habits:

- **Focus on foods first.** In HEED, we encourage you to focus on getting your nutrients from whole foods as opposed to getting them from pills and powders. You probably already know that foods provide many nutritional benefits, such as vitamins, minerals, and carbohydrate. But scientists have recently discovered additional components in foods, especially plant foods, that seem to provide health benefits. Food synergy—the ability of different components in foods to work together to enhance health—is another good reason to focus on foods. Besides, foods are fun to eat!

- **Believe that all foods can fit.** In HEED we emphasize eating a balanced diet of foods rich in nutrients. Still, we think that there is room in most people's diets for moderate amounts of foods that are less nutritious. In other words, we believe there's no such thing as "junk" food.

- **Make changes you can live with.** People are best able to maintain behavior changes if they make the changes gradually. We encourage you to be patient and not expect overnight results. Changing a habit is hard work!

- **Eat a balanced diet.** This is the key to reducing health risk factors and promoting health. Did you know your body needs more than 40 different nutrients to achieve and maintain good health? No single food or food group provides all the nutrients you need. You have to eat a variety of foods in appropriate amounts to get the important building blocks that keep your body healthy and strong. But what's the right balance? In this session we introduce a simple visual illustration that will help you make balanced food choices. Then you'll get to assess the nutritional balance of your own diet.

Let the Pyramid Be Your Guide

Our work and experience has focused on promoting dietary change in the United States. But we recognize that healthy eating is a growing international concern. Many diet-related diseases, such as obesity, diabetes, cancer, and cardiovascular disease, are on the rise worldwide. Thus, people in many English-speaking countries may be interested in using HEED to help them improve the quality of their diets. Throughout this book, we have included metric conversions and used some general terms that will be familiar to people in many countries. Where we couldn't find a general term that worked for most countries, we added footnotes to help explain the differences.

Many countries have developed dietary guidelines to reduce chronic diseases and promote health in their populations. Interestingly, most countries have similar dietary recommendations; they just have used different graphic designs to show people what they should be eating every day. For example, Canada uses a rainbow, Australia uses a plate, and the United States started using a pyramid in 1992. The Canadian rainbow, Australian plate, and American pyramid have been widely used in nutrition education programs, food packaging, and federal nutrition programs in each respective country.

Periodically, countries update their dietary recommendations based on new scientific findings. The United States federal government recently completed a major review and overhaul of its dietary guidelines. The recommendations released in 2005 focus on adopting a healthy eating pattern similar to the one we recommend in HEED. The 2005 guidelines recommend a diet that is high in fruits, vegetables, whole grains, and nonfat or low-fat dairy products and is low in saturated fats, cholesterol, and excess sugars. They also promote calorie balance. We have modified the previous American food pyramid and created our own HEED pyramid to reflect this new approach to healthy eating. Here's how we created the HEED pyramid (figure 1.2):

• Added physical activity as a daily goal. Physical activity is at the base of the HEED pyramid because it burns calories and helps you achieve or maintain a healthy weight. As with a healthy diet, regular physical activity provides many health benefits. How much physical activity do you get each day? The goal is to accumulate at least 30 minutes of moderate-intensity physical activity five or more days a week. We discuss the

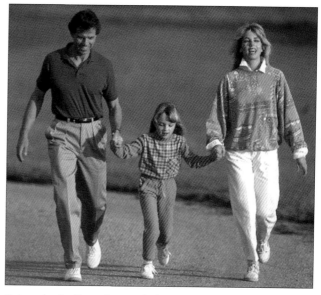

Being physically active can help you maintain or lose weight.

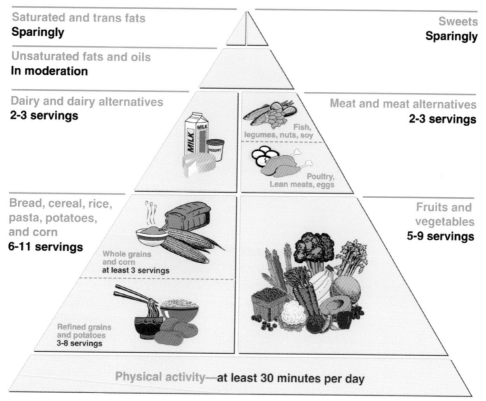

Saturated and trans fats
Sparingly

Unsaturated fats and oils
In moderation

Dairy and dairy alternatives
2-3 servings

Sweets
Sparingly

Meat and meat alternatives
2-3 servings

Fish, legumes, nuts, soy

Poultry, Lean meats, eggs

Bread, cereal, rice, pasta, potatoes, and corn
6-11 servings

Whole grains and corn
at least 3 servings

Refined grains and potatoes
3-8 servings

Fruits and vegetables
5-9 servings

Physical activity—**at least 30 minutes per day**

Figure 1.2 The Healthy Eating Every Day (HEED) pyramid.

Your Country's Dietary Guidelines

You can see various countries' dietary guidelines in session one of HEED Online. To enroll in HEED Online, go to www.ActiveLiving.info. You can read more about your country's food guidelines from these Web sites:

Canada

www.hc-sc.gc.ca

After choosing a preferred language, follow the "Healthy Living" link to the "Food & Nutrition" link and click on "Canada's Food Guide to Healthy Eating."

Australia

www.nhmrc.gov.au

Move your computer arrow over "Publications" to the left of the screen and then click on "Current Publications." When you see a list there, select "Nutrition" to view various publications on the dietary guidelines for adults, adolescents, and children.

New Zealand

www.healthed.govt.nz

In the "Health Topic" box, select "Nutrition" and click on "Search." You'll see a long list of links for many helpful nutrition publications. Select "Healthy Eating for Adult New Zealanders."

United Kingdom

www.wiredforhealth.gov.uk/doc.php?docid=7267

This Web page highlights nine guidelines for a healthy diet. It also offers suggestions on how to help achieve the guidelines.

role of physical activity as an integral part of a healthy lifestyle throughout this book.

- **Emphasized the need to eat more whole-grain bread group foods.** You'll notice that we have taken potatoes and corn out of the vegetables group and put them with the bread group foods. That's because their nutrient values are more like bread group foods than most other vegetables. We divided the bread, cereal, rice, pasta, sweet corn, and potatoes group into "refined grains and potatoes" and "whole grains and corn" because whole-grain foods are better sources of fiber, vitamins, and minerals than are refined grains and potatoes. Whole-grain foods are also good sources of phytochemicals, a new class of substances that scientists think may lower risk for cancer and heart disease. Plus, they are less likely than refined grains to cause spikes in blood sugar levels that may be linked to health problems such as diabetes and obesity. Even so, all bread group foods are part of the foundation of a healthy diet.

- **Combined the fruits and vegetables groups.** Both of these food groups are sources of similar nutrients, so they go well together. Also, we highlight the goal

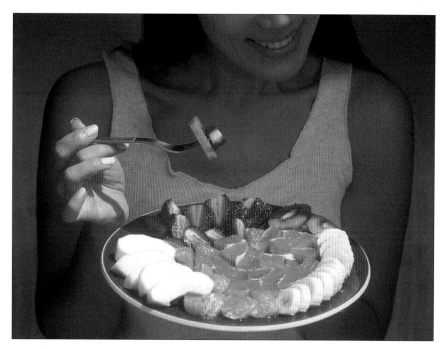

Fruits and vegetables are great sources of vitamins, minerals, fiber, and phytochemicals.

of five to nine daily servings of a variety of fruits and vegetables. This allows you more flexibility when choosing your fruits and vegetables. For example, one day you might eat three fruit and five vegetable servings. The next day you might eat one fruit and seven vegetable servings. As with whole-grain foods, fruits and vegetables are very rich sources of vitamins, minerals, fiber, and phytochemicals. Unfortunately, most adults do not get the recommended amount of fruits and vegetables each day, which means they are missing out on a lot of good nutrition.

❓ DID YOU KNOW?

Phyto-What?!?

Phytochemicals are substances other than vitamins and minerals that are found in plants and may protect our body's cells from the damaging effects of harmful substances. This in turn may reduce the risk of cancer and heart disease. We still have a lot to learn about the role of phytochemicals in health. But you can't go wrong by including a lot of whole grains and colorful fruits and vegetables in your diet. Plant foods, not supplements, are the best sources of these new nutrition wonders.

• **Divided the meat group into two subgroups.** All foods in these two subgroups are good sources of protein. Many are good sources of critical nutrients such as iron and zinc. The main difference between the two subgroups is the saturated fat and cholesterol content. Both saturated fat and cholesterol are known to raise blood cholesterol levels and can increase your risk for heart disease. Beef, pork, lamb, chicken, and eggs contain artery-clogging saturated fat and cholesterol. You can minimize the amount of these harmful substances by choosing lean meats, skinless poultry, and egg whites. On the other hand, fish, legumes, nuts, and soy foods are very low in saturated fats. Fish does contain cholesterol but usually in low to moderate amounts. In addition, fish, legumes, nuts, and soy foods are good sources of healthy fats and, except for fish, are good sources of fiber.

• **Included alternatives in the dairy group.** Dairy products (milk, yogurt, and cheese) are the best food sources of calcium. Calcium is important for bone health and may affect blood pressure and body weight. For health, ethical, or religious reasons, some people cannot eat dairy products that come from animals. Fortunately, there are many calcium-rich dairy alternatives, such as milk, yogurt, and cheese made from soy. You can even find dairy-free "milks" made from almonds, rice, and oats. When choosing a dairy alternative, be sure to select one that is fortified with calcium.

• **Divided "fats, oils, and sweets" into "unsaturated fats and oils," "saturated and trans fats," and "sweets."** These foods are at the tip of the pyramid because they should be eaten in smaller amounts than the other food groups. Although fats and oils should be a small part of the total diet, some are better than others. Unsaturated fats and oils provide important vitamins and fats that help reduce heart disease risk (table 1.1). Healthy oils include most vegetable oils, but especially canola, olive, and flaxseed oils. Soy, nuts, and fatty fish such as salmon, mackerel, and herring are also good sources of healthy oils. That's why these foods are excellent alternatives to meat and poultry. On the other hand, you could live just fine without eating any saturated and trans fats. These types of fats significantly raise blood cholesterol levels, which can increase heart disease risk. That's why foods that are high in these types of fats should be eaten sparingly. If they're available, select lower-fat options such as ground sirloin instead of regular ground beef.

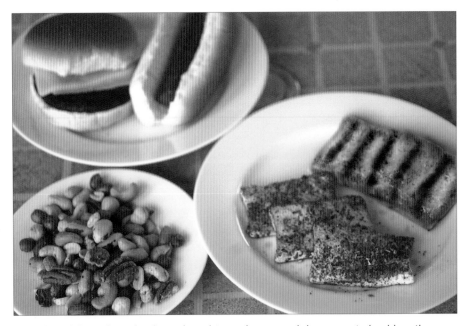

Nuts, fatty fish, and soy foods, such as this soy burger and dog, contain healthy oils.

The foods in the sweets category provide few nutrients but usually have a lot of calories. They are commonly called "empty-calorie" foods. You don't need to eat these foods very often. Many foods that are high in fat are also high in sugars—for example, pies, cakes, cookies,* and ice cream. Are you feeling doomed because you love sweet foods? Don't worry. These foods can fit into a healthy diet if eaten sparingly.

Table 1.1   Tale of Two Fat Categories

Foods high in unsaturated fats and oils	Foods high in saturated or trans fats
Health effect: Provide vitamin E, help maintain healthy blood cholesterol levels, and reduce risk of sudden death heart attack	*Health effect: Raise blood cholesterol levels*
Canola, olive, and flaxseed oils	Butter, lard, stick (hard) margarine, shortening
Corn, soybean, and cottonseed oils	Coconut, palm, and palm kernel oils
Fish oils	Hydrogenated or partially hydrogenated oils
Soybeans	Fried foods
Nuts	Commercially baked cakes, cookies,* crackers, and chips[†]
Salad dressings	Fatty cuts of meat, pork, lamb, lunch meats, bacon, and sausage
Liquid or tub margarine (soft margarine)	Whole and 2% milk
	Whole-milk cheese

*Same as *biscuits* in some countries.
[†]Same as *crisps* in some countries.

WEIGHTY MATTERS

How Sweet It Isn't

Most people in Western nations, adults and children alike, have a sweet tooth, no doubt about it. It is likely that the increase in foods high in sugar and other sweeteners has contributed to the obesity epidemic in many countries. Sweets by themselves don't cause disease. But eating highly sweetened foods adds very few nutrients and a lot of calories—something most people can ill afford. As with foods high in saturated and trans fats, you should limit your intake of sweetened foods:

- Chocolates or other sweet foods made from sugar
- Soft drinks and other sweetened beverages
- Cakes and cookies*
- Pies
- Sugar and honey
- Jam

*Same as *biscuits* in some countries.

? DID YOU KNOW?

Americans get about 25% of their daily calories from excess fats. That is, fats that they add while cooking or at the table and fats that come in foods that have lower-fat options (e.g., whole milk versus nonfat milk). An additional 15% of total calories comes from added sugars.[5] In England, added sugars account for about 13% of total daily calories.[6] If you can relate to these statistics, you might find that "decreasing fats" and "balancing calories" become some of your HEED goals.

Portions and Servings

The HEED pyramid recommends a certain number of daily *servings* of each food group. But what exactly is a *serving*? Many people think a serving is simply the *portion* of food they put on their plate. But that *portion* of pasta you put on your plate may actually be four to six *servings* of the bread group!

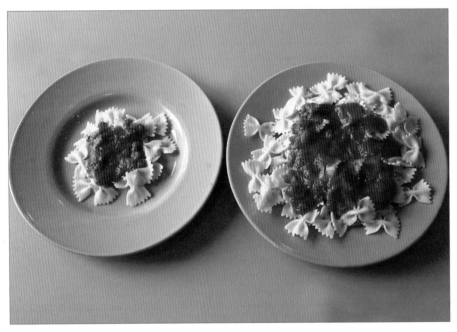

One serving of pasta is 1/2 cup or 70 g (one bread group serving), but many people eat closer to 3 cups or 420 g of pasta (six bread group servings).

It's very important that you learn the recommended serving sizes for each food group and match your *portions* (what you serve yourself) to the pyramid *servings* (the standard recommended amount). To help you in this process, we offer very specific guidelines for serving sizes in each food group (see page 11). See page 89 of session 7, too, for more on serving sizes.

? DID YOU KNOW?

According to a recent study,[7] foods commonly found in U.S. restaurants and stores have steadily increased in size since the 1970s. Today, the portion of chocolate chip cookies eaten is seven times the recommended serving size! Pasta portions exceed recommended amounts by nearly 500%. And bagels are about double the recommended serving amounts.

FOOD GROUP SERVING SIZES

Bread, Cereal, Rice, Pasta, Potatoes, and Corn

1 slice of bread

1/2 cup cooked cereal (120 g), rice (80 g), pasta (70 g), or corn (80 g)

1/2 cup (105 g) mashed potato

1 small (4-inch, 10-cm) potato

10 french fries*

1 ounce (30 g) ready-to-eat cereal (about 1 cup of flakes)

1/3 to 1/2 bagel or muffin

Fruits and Vegetables

1/2 cup (85 g) chopped raw, cooked, frozen, or canned fruit or vegetables

1 medium-sized piece of fruit or melon wedge

1 cup (55 g) leafy raw vegetables

3/4 cup (6 oz; 180 ml) fruit or vegetable juice

1/4 cup (35 g) dried fruit

Dairy and Dairy Alternatives

1 cup milk (240 ml) or yogurt (245 g)

1-1/2 ounces (45 g) natural cheese (such as cheddar)

2 ounces (60 g) of soy or processed cheese

1 cup (240 ml) soy milk or yogurt (245 g) with added calcium

Meat and Meat Alternatives

2-1/2 to 3 ounces (70-85 g) of cooked fish, poultry, or lean meat

Soy-based meat substitutes that have 18 to 25 grams of protein per serving

The following are equivalent to one ounce (28 g) of fish, poultry, or meat:

1/2 cup (90 g) cooked beans or tofu

1 egg

2 tbsp. of peanut butter or 1/3 cup (45 g) nuts

1/4 cup (65 g) tofu

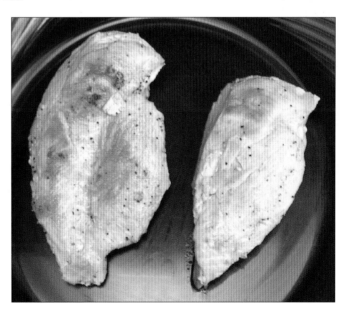

Compare the typical portion eaten (6 oz or 170 g) with one meat group serving of chicken (3 oz or 85 g).

*Also known as *chips* in some countries.

The Right Amount for *You*

Notice that the HEED pyramid recommends a *range* of servings for each food group. For example, a range of five to nine servings is recommended for the fruit and vegetable group. What's the right amount for you? Take a look at table 1.2 to find out.

People who need about 1,600 calories a day (most women and some older adults) should eat the lower number of the range for each food group. People who need about 2,200 calories a day (children, adolescent girls, and so on) should eat in about the middle of the serving range.

Someone who needs 2,000 calories a day should eat between the 1,600 and 2,200 calorie level. For example, they should eat seven servings of bread, six servings of fruits and vegetables, two servings of milk, and a total of six ounces (170 g) of meat.

Table 1.2   Recommended Servings for Different People

	Most women and some older adults	Children, adolescent girls, active women, and most men	Adolescent boys and active men
Caloric level	About 1,600	About 2,200	About 2,800
Bread group*	6	9	11
Fruit and vegetable group	5	7	9
Dairy group	2-3[†]	2-3[†]	2-3[†]
Meat group	2, for a total of 5 ounces (140 g)	2, for a total of 6 ounces (170 g)	3, for a total of 7 ounces (200 g)

*At least three servings should be whole-grain foods.

[†]Women who are pregnant or breastfeeding, teenagers, and young adults up to age 24 need three servings.

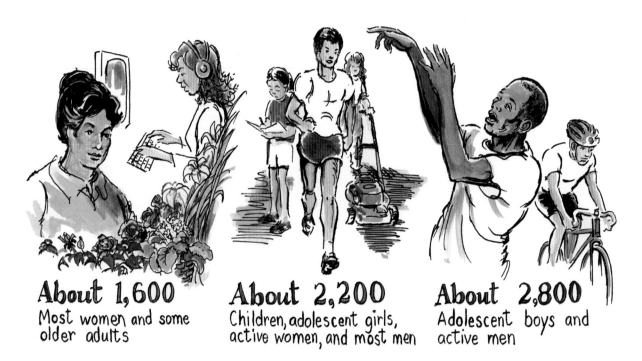

About 1,600
Most women and some older adults

About 2,200
Children, adolescent girls, active women, and most men

About 2,800
Adolescent boys and active men

To get a more precise estimate of your daily caloric needs and recommended servings in each food group, go to session 1 in HEED Online at www.ActiveLiving.info.

HEED Pyramid Assessment

We will often encourage you to record information about your eating habits, and this is the first instance. It is all right to write in this book. In fact, we've designed this book with that in mind. Feel free to write notes and to underline or highlight text that you find especially useful. Where we provide tables or blanks to write in, please do so!

How healthy do you think your diet is? People often think that their diet is healthier than it actually is. The best way to determine whether you're getting enough of the nutrients you need is to record what you eat in a day (choose a pretty typical day), and then count up the amounts of servings of each food group you consume. Follow these steps, recording your answers in table 1.3:

1. For one day, beginning with breakfast, write down everything you eat and drink. Include breakfast, lunch, dinner, and snacks. If your eating patterns are not that different from day to day, you can simply think back over yesterday's food intake and write it in the space provided.

2. For each food you listed, identify the amount you ate or typically eat. Measure the amounts, if possible.

3. For each food you listed, identify the food group it belongs to (e.g., fruits and vegetables) and translate the quantity you ate into pyramid *servings*. (Use the Food Group Serving Sizes on page 11.) For each food you listed, write the number of pyramid servings you ate in the column under the food group it belongs to. For instance, if you drank 6 ounces (180 ml) of orange juice at breakfast, you would write "1" under the fruits and vegetables column, because that represents one serving size of fruit.

4. The two fat groups and the sweets group require somewhat different treatment because there are no standard serving sizes for these groups.

   - Place a 1 in the unsaturated fats and oils column for each time you eat any of the foods listed in table 1.1, Tale of Two Fat Categories, on page 9.

   - Put a 1 in the saturated and trans fats category each time you eat butter, stick (hard) margarine, shortening, lard, whole milk dairy products, fatty meats, fried foods, and the like.

   - As with the fats categories, put a 1 in the sweets column every time you eat any amount of sweetened drinks, sweets,* sugar, honey, cake, cookies,† pie, and sweetened desserts.

5. Total the numbers in each group to view your daily intake.

Candy in the United States.
†Same as *biscuits* in some countries.

Table 1.3 My Daily Servings

Meal	Food eaten	Amount eaten	Bread, cereal, rice, pasta, potatoes, and corn	Servings eaten					Sweets occurrences
				Fruits and vegetables	Dairy and dairy alternatives	Meat and meat alternatives	Unsaturated fats and oils occurrences	Saturated and trans fats occurrences	
Breakfast									
Lunch									

Dinner													
Snacks													
Servings totals													

Now it's time to determine how your diet compares to what is recommended for you. To begin, transfer your daily serving totals from table 1.3 to the first column in table 1.4. Next, transfer your recommended servings from table 1.2 to the second column in table 1.4. Then calculate your pyramid needs by subtracting what is recommended for you from your actual intake and fill in that number in the third column in table 1.4. This shows you whether you are eating an appropriate amount of each food group.

- If you scored a zero, you are eating an appropriate amount of that food group.
- If you scored a positive number, you are eating too much of that food group.
- If you scored a negative number, you are eating too little of that food group.

Because there are no recommended servings for either of the fats categories, we have to treat these a little differently. Write your total intake for the unsaturated and saturated fat in table 1.5. Then subtract the saturated and trans fat category from the unsaturated oils. Your goal should be to end up with a positive number. In other words, you want to be eating more foods with "good" fats than foods with "bad" fats.

For the sweets group, enter your total intake from the sweets column of table 1.3 in the sweets row of table 1.5. Remember, the sweets category includes any food that contains added sugar, corn syrup, or honey. These foods have a lot of calories and few nutrients. You want to keep this number low, say to only one

Table 1.4   How Does My Diet Stack Up?

Food group	My daily servings	Recommended for me	Pyramid needs
Example: Fruit and vegetable group	3	5	-2
Bread group	_____	_____	_____
Fruit and vegetable group	_____	_____	_____
Dairy group	_____	_____	_____
Meat group	_____	_____	_____

Table 1.5   Oils, Fats, and Sweets Intake

	My intake		My intake
Unsaturated oils	_____	Sweets	_____
Saturated and trans fats	– _____		
Difference	_____		

or two per day. This is especially important if you are trying to manage your weight.

This simple assessment shows you where you need to balance your diet to make sure you are getting the nutrients you need for good health. You should now see which foods you are getting adequate amounts of, which you need more of, and which you need to eat less of. Record your results in the HEED Assessment Log in appendix A. Together with the HEED goals assessment that you will complete in session 2, you will get a good idea of the areas you need to work on to bring your diet into balance.

A Healthy Menu for Life

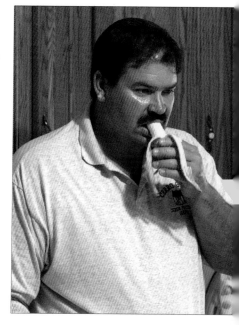

Making small changes toward healthy eating pays off in big ways. As we explained earlier, research has found that eating foods in line with the HEED pyramid eating pattern can reduce your risk of health problems.

What might a healthy menu look like? Take a look at the following balanced diet for someone needing about 2,000 calories per day.

Breakfast

1/2 cup (120 g) instant flavored oatmeal

1 mini whole-wheat bagel

1 medium banana

1 cup (240 ml) nonfat milk

1 tbsp. fat-free cream cheese

A banana can be part of a healthy breakfast.

Lunch

Chicken breast sandwich

- 3 ounces (85 g) skinless chicken breast
- 2 slices whole-wheat bread
- 1 slice reduced-fat cheese
- 1 large leaf lettuce
- 2 slices tomato
- 1 tbsp. low-fat mayonnaise

1 medium peach

1 cup (240 ml) apple juice

Dinner

3/4 cup (190 g) vegetarian spaghetti sauce

1 cup (140 g) pasta

3 tbsp. grated Parmesan cheese

Spinach salad

- 1 cup (30 g) fresh spinach leaves
- 1/4 cup (30 g) fresh grated carrots
- 1/4 cup (20 g) fresh mushrooms, sliced
- 2 tbsp. vinaigrette dressing

1/2 cup (80 g) cooked sweet corn

1/2 cup (120 g) canned pears, packed in fruit juice

Snacks

1/3 cup (45 g) almonds

1/4 cup (35 g) dried apricots

1 cup (245 g) fat-free fruit yogurt, no sugar added

Looks pretty good, doesn't it? The goal is for your daily menus to look similar. If this seems a little daunting to you—you can't imagine eating that many fruits and vegetables or not eating your usual amount of beef—stick with us! Over time, we'll show you small steps you can take to make your eating patterns healthier for a lifetime.

Three days of balanced menus for three different calorie levels (1,600; 2,200; and 2,800) are provided in session 1 of HEED Online at www.ActiveLiving.info.

Session Checklist

Before you move on to the next session's activities, be sure to do the following:

- Review the HEED pyramid.

- Think about how the portions you eat compare to the recommended serving sizes.

- Complete the HEED pyramid assessment, especially tables 1.3 to 1.5.

- Go to session 1 in HEED Online to get a personalized daily calorie and food group recommendation and to learn more about basic nutrition.

As you have seen in this session, healthy eating is a balancing act. You need a balance of foods from different food groups to ensure that you get all the nutrients your body needs. You need to balance the calories you eat with the calories your body uses to prevent weight gain. You also want to balance good nutrition with enjoying tasty and convenient foods. Like a gymnast learning a new routine on a balance beam, on some days you will do well balancing your diet and on others you will slip and fall off. As you learn more healthy eating skills in HEED, you will become better prepared to prevent slips and to get back on track if they happen. In the next session, you will complete the HEED goals assessment to determine the best place you can start improving your eating habits.

TWO

Taking Stock

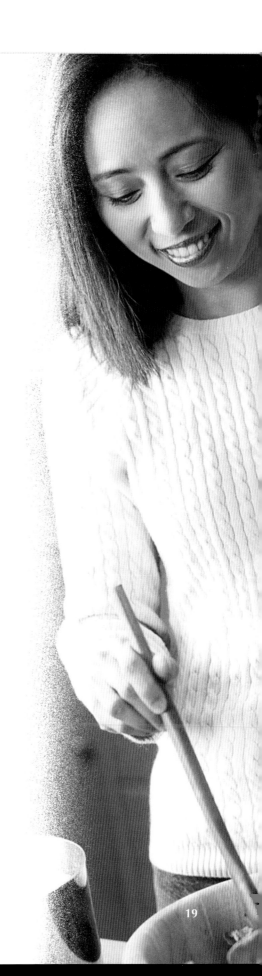

In This Session

- Assessing the health of your diet
- Understanding the five HEED goals
- Determining your readiness to change your eating habits

You've hit the ground running! Hopefully, you're excited about applying the HEED principles that you learned in session 1 to help you make changes to your eating habits. To assist you, we'll focus on five dietary changes that most people need to make. We've called these the five HEED goals. Right now you may need to only change one goal area. Or you may need help with all five and perhaps others in addition. No matter what shape your diet is in today, by the end of *Healthy Eating Every Day* (HEED) you'll have learned many skills and strategies to improve your eating habits and to maintain a healthy diet for a lifetime.

Don't worry if you feel a little overloaded with information. These first two sessions are the most difficult. During the next several weeks, you'll learn step-by-step strategies to put this knowledge to work for you. Let's keep your momentum going as you begin this important session! In this session, you'll assess your current eating habits and take a closer look at the five HEED goals. You'll also learn which areas of your diet you are more ready to change.

HEED Goals Assessment

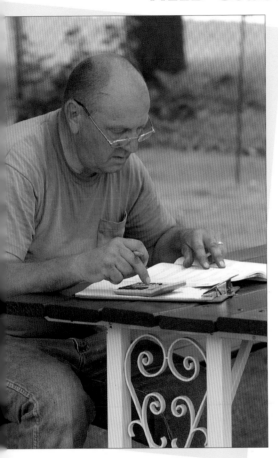

Up to this point we've explained the HEED approach to healthy eating and you've completed the HEED pyramid assessment. But before you can start to make healthy changes in your diet, you need to know more about how your diet compares to what is recommended. In the HEED goals assessment, you'll learn which areas of your diet you're doing best in and which areas need the most work. This will help you determine what area to focus on in the coming weeks. You'll have a chance to reassess your eating habits and update your goals several times throughout HEED.

The HEED goals assessment is not intended to precisely measure your dietary intake. It doesn't account for all factors—such as food allergies, frequency of meals, and social aspects—that may affect your eating choices. Rather, this assessment is designed to help you get a better sense of your specific habits in five important areas. Answer the questions as best you can, and don't worry if your score is a bit low. That's what HEED is here for—to help you improve your diet and your score!

The HEED goals assessment has five sections, with each section representing one of the five HEED goals. Complete this assessment of dietary habits by selecting one answer for each question. Be sure to read each answer carefully before choosing one. Note that a point value from 0 to 5 is associated with each answer. Write the score for each answer in the last column on the right. Then total the score for all questions at the bottom of each section. After each section of the assessment, you'll learn more about why this HEED goal area is important to a healthy diet.

Increasing Fruits and Vegetables

How often do you . . .

▥ Eat at least one serving of citrus fruit* (e.g., orange, grapefruit, lemon, or lime) or citrus fruit juice† per day?

0 points	1 point	3 points	5 points	Score
Rarely or never	1-3 times per week	4-5 times per week	6-7 times per week	_____

Eat at least one serving* of dark green, deep orange, yellow, or red fruits or vegetables per day?

0 points	1 point	3 points	5 points	Score
Rarely or never	1-3 times per week	4-5 times per week	6-7 times per week	_____

Choose fruits or vegetables as a snack instead of choosing a typical snack food?

0 points	1 point	3 points	5 points	Score
Rarely or never	1-3 times per week	4-5 times per week	6 or more times per week	_____

Try new ways to prepare, eat, or order fruits and vegetables?

0 points	1 point	3 points	5 points	Score
Rarely or never	1 time per month	2 times per month	3 or more times per month	_____

Select fruits or vegetables as side dishes when eating out?

0 points	1 point	3 points	5 points	Score
Rarely or never	1-2 times per month	3-4 times per month	5 or more times per month	_____

*1 serving = 1 medium-sized piece of fruit; 1/2 cup (85 g) chopped raw, cooked, frozen, or canned fruit or vegetables; 1/4 cup (35 g) dried fruit; 1 cup (55 g) leafy raw vegetables

[†]1 serving = 3/4 cup (6 oz; 180 ml) fruit or vegetable juice

Increasing Fruits and Vegetables Score (total) _____ out of 25

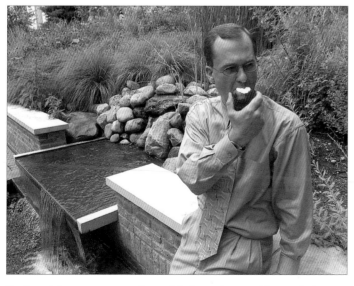

Try to eat five or more servings of fruits and vegetables each day.

It takes more than an apple a day to keep the doctor away. The goal is to eat at least five servings of fruits and vegetables every day. Eating more of these nutritional powerhouses is a simple way to boost your dietary balance. It's too bad that in the United States fewer than 30% of adults are eating the recommended number of fruit servings a day, and fewer than 60% are getting the recommended number of vegetable servings a day.[5] It's not just a problem in the United States. Adults in Great Britain average less than three servings of fruit and vegetables— well below the recommended level of five or more a day.[6]

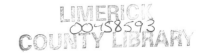

? DID YOU KNOW?

Why Vegetables?

Vegetables are very low in

- fat,
- calories, and
- cholesterol (actually, they have no cholesterol at all).

And they are rich in

- fiber,
- vitamins,
- minerals,
- antioxidants, and
- phytochemicals.

Decreasing Fats

Do you . . .

Use butter, margarine, or oils when cooking or as spreads?

0 points	3 points	5 points	Score
Usually choose butter, stick (hard) margarine, shortening, animal fat, or lard	Usually choose whipped or light (reduced-fat) butter or regular tub (soft) margarine	Usually choose liquid margarine, vegetable oils, or reduced-fat tub (soft) margarine	_____

Use salad dressing or mayonnaise?

0 points	3 points	5 points	Score
Usually choose regular option	Usually choose low-fat option	Usually choose nonfat option	_____

Eat beef, pork, lamb, or veal? (Give yourself five points if you rarely or never eat beef, pork, lamb, or veal.)

0 points	3 points	5 points	Score
Rarely choose lean cuts or lean ground* beef, and rarely remove excess fat before cooking or eating	Sometimes choose lean or extra-lean cuts or lean ground* beef, and sometimes remove excess fat before cooking or eating	Usually choose lean or extra-lean cuts or lean ground* beef, and usually remove excess fat before cooking or eating	_____

Eat turkey, chicken, or other poultry? (Give yourself five points if you rarely or never eat any type of poultry.)

0 points	3 points	5 points	Score
Usually choose fried poultry cooked with skin (and you eat the skin) or regular ground* poultry	Sometimes choose baked, broiled, or grilled poultry; poultry cooked with skin (but you don't eat the skin) or lean ground* poultry	Usually choose baked, broiled, or grilled poultry; poultry cooked and eaten without skin; or lean ground* poultry	_____

Eat fish, shellfish, or seafood?

0 points	3 points	5 points	Score
Usually choose fried fish	Sometimes choose fried fish	Usually choose baked, broiled, or grilled fish	_____

Eat cheese?

0 points	3 points	5 points	Score
Usually choose regular option	Sometimes choose low-fat option	Usually choose nonfat or low-fat option	_____

Choose the light or low-fat version of foods and sauces when available?

0 points	1 point	3 points	5 points	Score
Rarely or never	1-3 times per week	4-5 times per week	6 or more times per week	_____

Use the following preparation methods?

0 points	3 points	5 points	Score
Usually fry or saute	Sometimes bake, broil, steam, or grill	Usually bake, broil, steam, or grill	_____

Decreasing Fat Score (total) _____out of 40

The most recent dietary recommendations allow up to 35% of total calories as fat. U.S. national surveys show that the average American adult consumes about 33% of total calories as fat.[8] It is about the same in Australia and slightly higher (35%) in Great Britain. Hooray! Still, as you'll learn in HEED, most people need to concentrate on reducing certain *types* of fat, particularly saturated and trans fats. But fat adds flavor to foods, so we don't want you to become a fat fanatic!

*Also referred to as *minced* in some countries.

Increasing Dairy and Dairy Alternatives

How often do you . . .

Drink milk or soy milk?

0 points	1 point	3 points	5 points	Score
Rarely or never	1-6 times per week	1 time per day (7 times per week)	2 or more times per day	_____

Eat yogurt or soy yogurt?

0 points	1 point	3 points	5 points	Score
Rarely or never	1-6 times per week	1 time per day (7 times per week)	2 or more times per day	_____

Eat natural or processed cheese or soy cheese (cubed, sliced, or shredded)?

0 points	1 point	3 points	5 points	Score
Rarely or never	1-3 times per week	4-5 times per week	6 or more times per week	_____

Eat soft cheeses such as cottage cheese or ricotta cheese?

0 points	1 point	3 points	5 points	Score
Rarely or never	1-3 times per week	4-5 times per week	6 or more times per week	_____

Eat calcium-fortified foods or drinks such as orange juice, cereal, tofu, bread, or pasta?

0 points	1 point	3 points	5 points	Score
Rarely or never	1-3 times per week	4-5 times per week	6 or more times per week	_____

Increasing Dairy and Dairy Alternatives Score (total) _____ out of 25

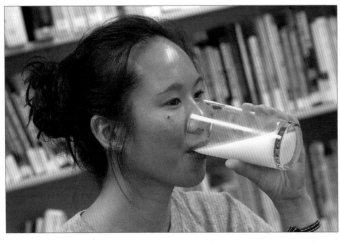

Try to eat or drink two to three servings of dairy products per day.

How are you doing with the assessment? Have some of your scores surprised you? Don't be too surprised if you scored really low in the dairy group. Most people do. But milk, yogurt, and other milk-based products are the best dietary sources of calcium. Before you decide to get the calcium you need from a calcium supplement, realize that dairy foods provide other important nutrients. Dairy products supply phosphorous and in many cases vitamin D, both of which are essential for bone health. Also, research suggests that eating dairy foods may help lower blood pressure and even body weight. This is not simply due to their calcium content.

What Is Lactose Intolerance?

Many people avoid milk and other dairy foods because they are lactose intolerant, a condition in which people find it difficult to digest lactose, the natural sugar found in milk and milk products. That's because they have too little of an enzyme called lactase. The undigested lactose sugar is used as food by the intestine's healthy bacteria, which then produce a gas that causes bloating, nausea, cramping, or diarrhea.

If you have been diagnosed with or suspect that you have lactose intolerance, it doesn't mean that you have to give up the wonderful health benefits of dairy products. In fact, most people with lactose intolerance are able to consume some milk products each day. Here are some tips:

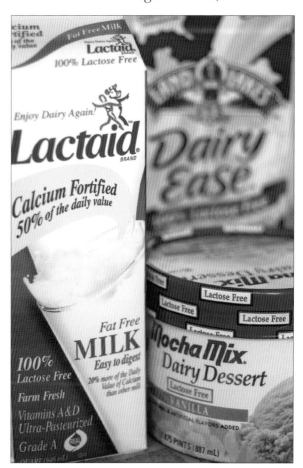

You should be able to find many lactose-free and lactose-reduced dairy products.

- Use lactose-reduced or lactose-free milk and milk products.

- Get a lactase supplement (ask your pharmacist). This is an over-the-counter pill containing lactase. You simply take a pill before eating milk products.

- Eat milk products with other foods as part of a meal or snack instead of eating them by themselves.

- Eat milk products in smaller amounts than the usual portion throughout the day.

- Try different dairy products. Some cheeses and some yogurts contain very small amounts of lactose.

- Calcium-fortified soy products can be good, lactose-free alternatives.

- If all else fails, add a calcium supplement with vitamin D to your daily routine. Aim for 500 to 1,000 milligrams of calcium and 400 of vitamin D. This will ensure that you're getting the bone-strengthening calcium that you need.

Increasing Whole Grains

How often do you . . .

Eat at least three servings* of whole-grain foods per day?

0 points	1 point	3 points	5 points	Score
Rarely or never	1-3 times per week	4-5 times per week	6-7 times per week	_____

Eat whole-grain ready-to-eat or hot cereal?

0 points	1 point	3 points	5 points	Score
Rarely or never	1-3 times per week	4-5 times per week	6 or more times per week	_____

Eat whole-wheat bread or rolls for sandwiches, toast, or at meals?

0 points	1 point	3 points	5 points	Score
Rarely or never	1-3 times per week	4-5 times per week	6 or more times per week	_____

Eat whole-grain pasta, brown rice, or other whole-grain side dishes?

0 points	1 point	3 points	5 points	Score
Rarely or never	1-3 times per week	4-5 times per week	6 or more times per week	_____

Eat popcorn or whole-grain snacks?

0 points	1 point	3 points	5 points	Score
Rarely or never	1-3 times per week	4-5 times per week	6 or more times per week	_____

Eat whole-grain foods that you haven't tried before?

0 points	1 point	3 points	5 points	Score
Rarely or never	1 time per month	2 times per month	3 or more times per month	_____

*1 serving = 1 slice of bread; one 6-inch tortilla; 1 ounce (30 g, or about 1 cup) ready-to-eat cereal; 1/2 cup cooked cereal (120 g), pasta (70 g), rice (80 g), or sweet corn (80 g)

Increasing Whole Grains Score (total) _____out of 30

The average adult barely eats one serving a day of whole-grain foods.[9] Is this you? Whole grains are rich sources of dietary fiber, carbohydrate, and phytochemicals that may help reduce risk for cancer and heart disease. Because they are more filling than foods made from refined grains, they may also be helpful in reducing daily caloric intake.

Balancing Calories

How often do you . . .

▦ Read food labels to see how many calories are in foods?

0 points	1 point	3 points	5 points	Score
Rarely or never	1-3 times per week	4-5 times per week	6 or more times per week	_____

▦ Track your daily caloric intake by writing down what you eat or by keeping track in your head?

0 points	1 point	3 points	5 points	Score
Rarely or never	1-3 days per week	4-5 days per week	6-7 days per week	_____

▦ Adjust how much you eat based on the amount of physical activity or exercise you get each day?

0 points	1 point	3 points	5 points	Score
Rarely or never	1-3 times per week	4-5 times per week	6 or more times per week	_____

▦ Make an effort to limit your portion sizes?

0 points	1 point	3 points	5 points	Score
Rarely or never	1-3 times per week	4-5 times per week	6 or more times per week	_____

▦ Choose low-calorie foods and beverages when available?

0 points	1 point	3 points	5 points	Score
Rarely or never	1-3 times per week	4-5 times per week	6 or more times per week	_____

▦ Eat when you are not hungry?

0 points	1 point	3 points	5 points	Score
6 or more times per week	4-5 times per week	1-3 times per week	Rarely or never	_____

Balancing Calories Score (total) _____ out of 30

Gaining weight is the simple result of eating more calories than your body needs. The extra calories get stored as body fat. Given the epidemic of obesity that has gripped most developed countries in the last three decades, a lot of people need to better balance their caloric intake (what they eat) with their caloric expenditure (how much physical activity they get). If you struggle in this area, you'll be interested in the Weighty Matters sidebars we've included throughout this book.

WEIGHTY MATTERS

Healthy Eating Every Day is not designed to be a restrictive weight-loss program. However, by heeding our advice, you may lose some weight if you are overweight. If you're not overweight, the dietary approach we recommend will help you win the battle of the bulge as you grow older. That's because you'll become more aware of the calories in the foods you're eating, learn about realistic portions, reduce your fat intake, boost your intake of fiber-rich foods, and begin to get moving. You'll also learn the life-management skills that will help make these changes stick.

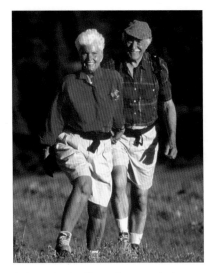

Being physically active can help you balance your calories.

Just how much can healthy eating patterns help you prevent weight gain? One recent study followed a group of normal weight, middle-aged women for an average of 12 years. Some of these women ate a diet similar to what we recommend in HEED. They ate a diet high in fruits, vegetables, low-fat milk, and other low-fat and high-fiber foods. Other women in the study ate more empty-calorie snacks, sweetened beverages, and sweets rich in fats. This second group also ate fewer fruits, vegetables, and other fiber-rich foods. They were 40% more likely to become overweight in the follow-up period than the group that ate the healthier diet.[10]

Although the focus of HEED is on healthy eating, we recognize that many people want to better manage their weight. That's why one of the HEED goals is to help you balance calories. That's also why we include a Weighty Matters segment in most of the sessions. We'll focus entirely on weight management in session 15.

Healthy Eating Every Day Score

Now that you've evaluated the different parts of your diet, transfer your total scores for each goal area to the space provided. Add all of your scores to get your grand total.

Increasing fruits and vegetables   _____ out of 25

Decreasing fats   _____ out of 40

Increasing dairy and dairy alternatives   _____ out of 25

Increasing whole grains   _____ out of 30

Balancing calories   _____ out of 30

Grand total   _____ out of 150

What Your Score Means

Compare your total score with the following categories. This is your starting point in HEED. You'll get to reassess your eating habits at the midpoint of the program and during the last session. This will help you see in what areas you have made improvements, in what areas you have slipped back a little, and how you are doing overall. To help you keep track of your scores throughout HEED, turn to appendix A and fill in the HEED Assessment Log with today's date and your scores.

115-150	Excellent! You are making many healthy food choices. Still, you may need to improve a little in some areas. Did you score much lower in any of the five goal areas compared to the others? If so, look to see what it would take to increase your score in that area. Did you score a 0, 1, or 3 on any of the questions? If so, those are specific areas you can work on in HEED.
85-114	You're on the right track, but you could do better. Review the different food habits within each goal area and pick four to six that you will be willing to work on in HEED. Think about what it would take for you to earn all fives within each goal area. The skills you'll learn in the HEED program will help you achieve these goals.
55-84	Congratulate yourself for making some healthy food choices. But to get the full benefits of healthy eating, you'll need to improve your eating habits. HEED can help. Take a look at the two goal areas in which you scored the lowest. These may be good places to start changing your diet.
Less than 55	Roll up your shirtsleeves. Your diet needs a lot of work and may be putting you at an increased risk of health problems. Don't try to change everything at once. HEED will show you many tips and strategies for improving the quality of your diet. Pick one or two goal areas to start with. You'll have plenty of time to work on other areas later.

We hope you found the HEED pyramid assessment in session 1 and the HEED goals assessment in this session helpful. By completing both assessments, you've learned a lot about your eating habits. You may be wondering why you had to complete *two* separate assessments. The purpose of the pyramid assessment is to determine if you're getting the recommended number of servings in each of the HEED food groups and getting a good balance of foods. The HEED goals assessment provides more detail on the type of choices you are making in the five HEED goal areas. In the weeks to come, use these two assessments to help you determine which areas of your diet need the most improvement.

Don't be discouraged if you have a lot of work to do. And be careful about being overconfident if your diet rates pretty highly. Hectic schedules and major life changes, such as marriage, relocation, a new job, and other demands, have a way of knocking even the best eaters off track. In either case, HEED provides you with the best available tools to help you learn how to change to—or maintain—a healthy diet for a lifetime.

Making Changes

Changing habits can be hard. How many times have you made a pact with yourself to improve your diet, lose weight, begin exercising, or spend more time with the people you love? You convince yourself each time that it will be different, that you will succeed. Usually you do succeed . . . for a while, and then other things take your attention and you forget your goal. Often you're left feeling like a failure. But you're not! In most cases, you were simply not ready to change.

Stages of Change

For decades, researchers have been studying what it takes for people to change health habits. What we have learned is that people go through different stages of readiness to change. Specific skills help people to move through the different stages. Researchers have examined the change process in people who quit smoking, stopped gambling, started exercising, or improved their diets. They've found that the five stages of readiness to change are these:

Precontemplation → Contemplation → Preparation → Action → Maintenance

Precontemplators aren't even thinking of changing a health habit. Perhaps it's because they don't know they should, or maybe they tried in the past but didn't succeed. **Contemplators** are thinking about making changes but haven't done anything to really change. These people may know some of the benefits of changing but don't know how to get started. People in the **preparation** stage have been trying to adopt a new habit but have not been able to be consistent. They may seek out information on how to change or may even try the new habit, but they usually don't stick with it more than a few days. People in the **action** stage

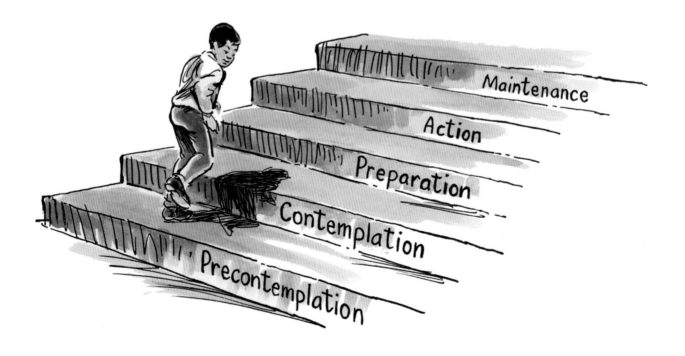

are successfully sticking with the new habit; they just haven't continued it for a long time. We define "a long time" as six months or even longer for some people. As you might have guessed, **maintainers** have maintained the habit for more than six months. Maintainers have learned the skills and strategies that it takes for them to keep doing the new behavior—so much so that it has become a new habit! And the new habit is something they value as important. It's very likely that a maintainer will do the new habit regardless of the barriers or roadblocks that occur in the future.

People don't arrive at the maintenance stage overnight. It takes time, trial and error, and a lot of patience to truly make the new habit last a lifetime. In fact, as you move through the stages of readiness, you are likely to move forward and backward. Every move, forward or backward, is part of the normal learning process. **Lapses are not signs of failure; they are signs that you are trying!**

For example, you may stay in the contemplation stage for a long time before you move to a new stage. You may move through the preparation stage quickly but then stay in action for only a short time before a minor problem causes you to move back to contemplation or preparation. This is not a sign of failure; it's a sign that you are trying.

Different Habits, Different Stages

Healthy Eating Every Day focuses on helping people improve their diets in five areas—fruits and vegetables, fats, dairy products and dairy alternatives, whole grains, and calories. It's very likely that you are in different stages of readiness for each of these dietary components. You can use the Am I Ready? form on page 33 to find out how ready you are to change your eating habits in each goal area.

UP CLOSE AND PERSONAL

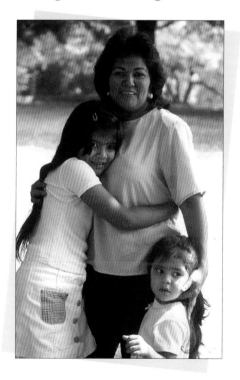

Meet Teri, a 42-year-old stay-at-home mother of two. Teri stopped drinking milk once she reached 18. She figured she wasn't growing any more, so she didn't need it. She doesn't eat a lot of cheese or yogurt because she thinks they have a lot of fat. Teri is trying to lose weight, so she mostly drinks diet soft drinks or coffee for beverages as a way of cutting back on her calories. Teri grew up in a household that never ate whole grains. In fact, she doesn't even know what counts as a whole grain. As a frequent dieter, she has learned how to keep her fat intake low and has recently increased her intake of fruits and vegetables to five servings a day. This is how Teri filled out the Am I Ready? form.

(continued)

(continued)

Am I Ready? (Teri's Form)

HEED dietary goals	Stage of readiness to change				
	Precontempla-tion (P)	Contemplation (C)	Preparation (PP)	Action (A)	Maintenance (M)
	I am not intend-ing to do this	I am not cur-rently doing this, but I have been thinking about working on it	I am doing this on some days each week but not every day	I am doing this successfully, but I have been doing it for less than six months	I have been doing this suc-cessfully for six months or more
Increase fruits and vegetables to at least 5 daily servings				✓	
Decrease fat intake by choos-ing lean, low-fat, and nonfat foods most of the time					✓
Increase dairy and dairy alter-natives to at least 2 daily servings	✓				
Increase whole grains to at least 3 daily servings	✓				
Balance calories (by balancing caloric intake and physical activity)			✓		

Teri is already in the maintenance stage for reducing fat in her diet. She is in the action stage for increasing fruits and vegetables. But she is in precontempla-tion for eating whole-grain foods and dairy products. She's in preparation for balancing calories. Which area do you think would be a good place for her to start working on her diet? If you said balancing calories, you're right. She's already made healthy changes by decreasing fats and increasing fruits and vegetables, and she is more ready to balance her calories than to increase her whole grains or dairy foods. ∎

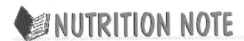 **NUTRITION NOTE**

Assessing My Readiness to Change

Now it's your turn. For each of the five dietary goal areas that are shown in the left-hand column of the table, select *one* of the categories across the top that best describes your readiness to change. Be sure to only choose one stage for each dietary goal.

Am I Ready?

HEED dietary goals	Stage of readiness to change				
	Precontempla-tion (P)	Contemplation (C)	Preparation (PP)	Action (A)	Maintenance (M)
	I am not intending to do this	I am not cur-rently doing this, but I have been thinking about working on it	I am doing this on some days each week but not every day	I am doing this successfully, but I have been doing it for less than six months	I have been doing this suc-cessfully for six months or more
Increase fruits and vegetables to at least 5 daily servings					
Decrease fat intake by choosing lean, low-fat, and nonfat foods most of the time					
Increase dairy and dairy alternatives to at least 2 daily servings					
Increase whole grains to at least 3 daily servings					
Balance calories (by balancing caloric intake and physical activity)					

From *Healthy Eating Every Day,* by Ruth Ann Carpenter and Carrie E. Finley, 2005, Champaign, IL: Human Kinetics. Organizations and agencies may not photocopy any material for professional or organizational use or distribution.

Why is this information important? Knowing the stage you are in for each goal area gives you a better idea of where you should focus your efforts. We'll discuss this further in the next session. For now, turn to appendix A and record your stage of readiness to change for each HEED goal in the HEED Assessment Log. Circle the letter in appendix A that matches your selections in the form above. You'll return to this form periodically to record any changes you make in your readiness to change.

Strategies for Change

Of course, the ultimate goal is to be in the maintenance stage for all five HEED dietary goals. But how do you move from one stage to the next? That's what we will be discussing in the rest of this book. Research has shown that people who use the following strategies are likely to succeed in changing their habits.

- Tracking daily habits
- Knowing your barriers and your benefits
- Setting realistic goals
- Rewarding yourself
- Recruiting help from friends and family
- Asserting yourself

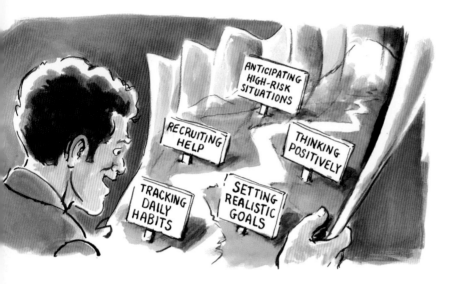

- Thinking positively
- Reminding yourself
- Anticipating high-risk situations
- Managing stress

From our physical activity studies we have learned that people who use these strategies are more likely to be doing the recommended amount of exercise after two years. We believe the same strategies are important for people who want to adopt healthy eating habits. During the next several sessions you'll learn more about these strategies and how to use them to help you achieve your healthy eating goals! We'll also share with you other skills such as managing portion sizes, healthy shopping and cooking, and eating out in healthy ways. All of these skills will help you make eating a balanced diet a lifelong habit.

Session Checklist

Before you move on to the next session's activities, be sure to do the following:

- ▪ Complete the HEED goals assessment.

- ▪ Complete the Am I Ready? form.

- ▪ Go to session 2 in HEED Online for more information about how diet affects your health.

Phew! These first two sessions have been pretty intense. We have asked you to do a lot of thinking, calculating, and recording. You'll be glad to know that few of the sessions in the future will be as demanding. As with most things in life, your success in HEED will be determined by the effort you put into it. You should now have a better idea of why and how you should improve your eating habits. In upcoming sessions, we'll help you develop skills to bring your diet into balance. These skills will help you stick with the changes that you make for a lifetime. Although the science of nutrition is very complex, the art of eating right is simple, especially when you know what areas of your diet need to be improved.

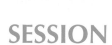

THREE

Setting Goals and Rewarding Yourself

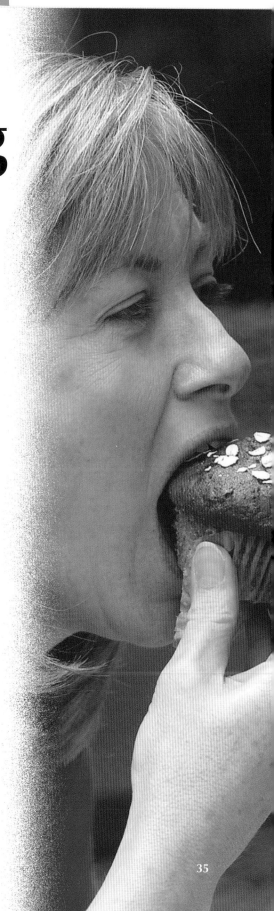

In This Session

- Learning the four characteristics of effective goals

- Setting effective long-term and short-term goals and rewards

- Learning the important skill of self-monitoring

Yeah, yeah, yeah. You've heard it before. People who set goals are more successful at making changes. But if it's so important, why can so few people recite their personal or professional goals? Often they just don't take time to think about their goals. Perhaps they don't know how to set *good* goals. Or maybe they don't reward themselves for attaining their goals, so reaching a goal isn't fun. Sound familiar? This session gives you a chance to focus on setting effective healthy eating goals—and rewarding yourself! As with other skills you will learn in HEED, setting good goals and rewarding your positive behavior are essential ingredients in a lifetime of healthy eating. The last part of the session introduces you to the important skill of self-monitoring. Self-monitoring will help you see if you're staying on track to meet your goals.

Elements of an Effective Goal

Take a look at these goals set by some of the participants in our nutrition research studies:

- "My doctor wants me to eat more whole grains."
- "I am going to lose 50 pounds (23 kg) in three months."
- "I will drink fewer soft drinks this week."
- "I will eat more fruits and vegetables this week."

If these were your healthy eating goals, is it likely that you would be able to achieve them? Probably not. That's because each of these goals is missing one or more of the core elements that make up a good goal. A goal has to be *personal, reasonable, specific,* and *measurable.* Let's look at each of these elements more closely.

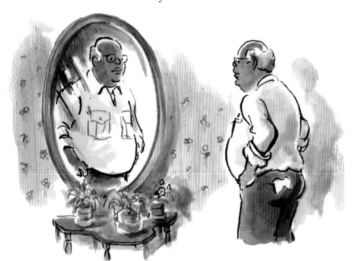

Personal. You're not likely to be successful in accomplishing your goals if they are set by someone other than yourself, such as a spouse, your doctor, or a co-worker. Personal goals are the goals that *you* believe in and truly want to achieve.

Bad example: My doctor wants me to eat more whole grains.

Good example: I have learned that eating whole grains is important to reducing my diabetes risk, so I will eat an average of three whole-grain servings per day for the next four weeks.

Realistic. We all want to do wonderful things, but our goals have to be reasonable and attainable. It's OK to push yourself, but you also must look objectively at yourself when deciding if a goal is realistic. In fact, studies show that if you set a challenging but realistic goal, you'll increase your performance better than if you set a goal that is too easy to attain.

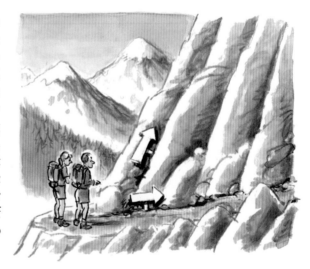

Bad example: I am going to lose 50 pounds (23 kg) in three months.

Good example: I will lose 6 to 12 pounds (3.0 to 5.5 kg) in three months. (Many health professionals recommend a weight loss of 1/2 to 1 pound, or 0.25 to 0.5 kilograms, per week. You're more likely to sustain this weight loss over time.)

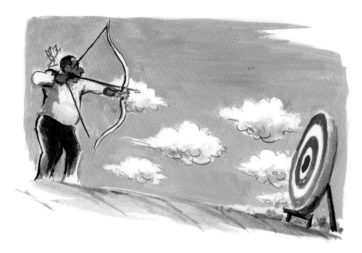

Specific. You need to clearly define what you intend to do or achieve. That means stating a clear and concise objective of what is to be accomplished. You'll need to prioritize steps, organize plans, and establish a timeline for reaching your goal. Vague statements about what you hope to achieve will leave you wondering what you wanted to accomplish.

Bad example: I will drink fewer soft drinks this week.

Good example: I will limit myself to one 12-ounce (355-ml) serving of a regular soft drink per day on Monday, Wednesday, and Friday.

Measurable. After you have laid the groundwork of choosing a personal, realistic, and specific goal, you need to state how you will know whether you have achieved your goal. This makes you accountable to yourself. Concluding each goal with a clause that says, "as confirmed by _____" can do this. You would fill in the blank with a plan for assessing whether you met the goal. You should periodically review your goals and evaluate them to see if you are staying on target.

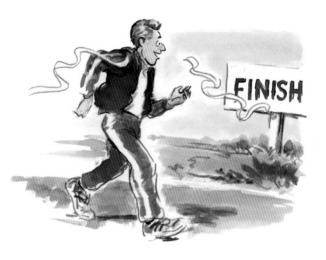

Bad example: I will eat more fruits and vegetables this week.

Good example: In the coming week, I will eat at least five servings of fruits and vegetables on Monday, Tuesday, Thursday, Friday, and Saturday *as confirmed by recording my food intake in my daily planner.*

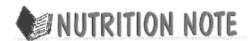 NUTRITION NOTE

Test Yourself

Do you know a good goal when you see it? Here's a chance to test yourself. For each of the following goal statements, see if you can identify whether it is a good goal or needs something changed to become a good goal. Remember, you want to determine whether the goal is personal, realistic, specific, and measurable. (Answers are on page 40.)

Example: "My doctor says that I need to lose some weight."

Not personal, specific, or measurable.

1. I will eat more dairy or calcium-rich foods.

2. During the next two weeks, I will eat at least two servings of dairy foods on five of the seven days by having milk for breakfast and yogurt as a snack as confirmed by my food log.

3. I will lose 15 pounds (6.8 kg) next week.

4. I will seek out restaurants that have healthy food as confirmed by my food records.

5. My spouse wants me to eat more salads on the weekends.

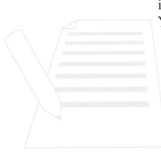 SCIENCE UPDATE

We noted earlier that people who set good goals are more likely to be successful in changing their habits. In a four-week study done at the City University of New York, 139 participants were assigned to one of four groups:[11]

1. Set goals to increase fiber intake by 5 grams per week up to the public health goal of 25 to 35 grams per day
2. Kept daily records of fiber intake
3. Set goals and kept records
4. Did not set goals or keep records

At the end of the study, the average fiber intake of the two groups that set goals (groups 1 and 3) was nearly double that of the other two groups. ▌

The Long and Short of It

Now that you know the four elements of effective goals, it's time for you to think about two types of goals. *Long-term goals* usually represent a pretty big change from where you are today, so they often require some time to reach them, say a month or longer. For example, a long-term goal could be, "At the end of three months, I will be eating breakfast on at least five days per week as confirmed by my food log." For a breakfast skipper, this would be a big change that might require smaller steps to achieve. These smaller steps would lend themselves to short-term goals. *Short-term goals* are smaller goals that you can accomplish in less than a month. For example, "In the next two weeks, I will eat breakfast at home on Mondays, Wednesdays, and Thursdays as confirmed by my daily food log." You can see how a succession of short-term goals can lead to the attainment of a long-term goal.

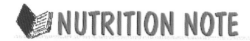 **NUTRITION NOTE**

Ready? Set Goals!

So here's your chance to take a step toward improving the quality of your diet. First, review the scores that you recorded in the HEED Assessment Log in appendix A. Remember that both the HEED pyramid assessment and the HEED goals assessment provide valuable information about your current eating habits. By reviewing your assessment scores you can see which HEED pyramid or HEED goal area needs the most improvement. Also keep in mind which area you are most *ready* to change.

Think of one or two long-term healthy eating goals that you want to reach. Write them in the space provided. Try to focus your goals on one or two specific HEED areas in which you need improvement and in which you're ready to change. Skip the rewards sections for now.

My Long-Term Goals (one month or longer)

Example: Within two months, I will be eating three servings of fruit per day as confirmed by my daily food log.

Goal 1: _____

_____

Reward: _____

Goal 2: _____

_____

Reward: _____

Now think of the short-term goals that you will need to attain to reach your long-term goals. You might have several short-term goals for each long-term goal. Remember the rules of good goal setting: Good goals are personal, reasonable, specific, and measurable. Again, skip the rewards sections for now.

(continued)

My Short-Term Goals (less than one month)

Example: By next Friday, I will have included at least one serving of fruit with each breakfast,

as confirmed by notes in my daily food log.

Goal 1: _____

_____

Reward: _____

Goal 2: _____

_____

Reward: _____

Goal 3: _____

_____

Reward: _____

Goal 4: _____

_____

Reward: _____

Setting personal, realistic, specific, and measurable goals isn't an easy task. But accomplishing these goals can be even more difficult. Lucky for you, we've provided a list of tips and strategies in appendix C for how to meet your goals in the five HEED goal areas. Use this list as a springboard to get you started on your way. Several sessions of HEED Online (accessed through www.ActiveLiving.info) contain even more strategies for accomplishing your goals.

Test Yourself Answer Key

1. The goal is not specific or measurable.

2. The goal is good—it's personal, realistic, specific, and measurable.

3. The goal is unrealistic. A realistic weight loss is 1/2 to 1 pound (0.23 to 0.45 kg) per week.

4. The goal is personal and realistic, but it is not specific enough to be measurable.

5. The goal is realistic, but it is not personal, specific, or measurable.

Your Just Rewards

We all like to be recognized or rewarded for a job well done at home, work, or in the community. When it comes to changing eating habits, rewards help us stay enthusiastic and focused on reaching our goals. They can be used for achieving both short-term and long-term goals. Rewards can be tangible things such as getting a massage, buying a new CD, going to the movies, attending a concert or sporting event, buying a new kitchen utensil, consulting with a dietitian, or going on a weekend getaway. Other rewards are intangible. That is, you cannot see, touch, or buy them. Rewarding yourself with self-praise, relaxing in a bubble bath, allowing yourself time to read the entire Sunday newspaper, taking your child to the zoo, and spending the afternoon relaxing with your spouse are examples of intangible rewards.

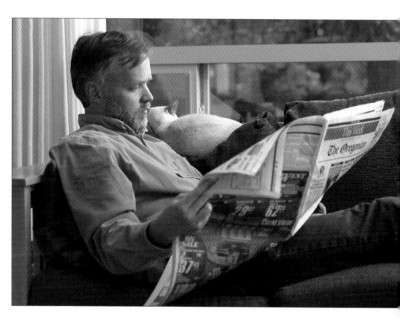

You can reward yourself by purchasing a gift for yourself or by taking time to read a newspaper.

NUTRITION NOTE

My Rewards

How would you like to reward yourself for eating better? Write down a list of incentives—large and small, tangible and intangible—that you would find rewarding. Be creative!

Tangible rewards

_____

_____

Intangible rewards

_____

_____

(continued)

(continued)

Tangible rewards	**Intangible rewards**
_____	_____
_____	_____
_____	_____

As you consider potential rewards, try to focus on those that are not food related but still bring you enjoyment. If you do choose a food reward, make it consistent with your goals for overall dietary improvement. For example, you might treat yourself to a small serving of your favorite low-fat dessert.

Now go back to your long- and short-term goals on pages 39 and 40 and add a reward for each one. Be careful to match the size of the reward to the size of the goal. For example, if you achieve your goal of eating three servings of fruits per day for a week, you wouldn't reward yourself with a trip to Hawaii! Perhaps a more appropriate reward might be to buy yourself a new shirt or a kitchen item, such as an apple peeler.

UP CLOSE AND PERSONAL

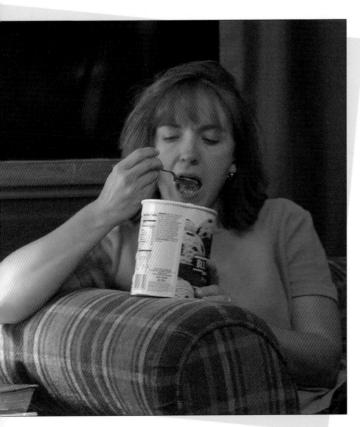

Sarah has worked for 15 years as a social worker. Her job is very stressful and draining. High case loads, heart-wrenching personal sagas, and relatively low pay contribute to high burnout rates for people in her profession. Sarah has staved off major burnout by setting goals in her professional and personal lives. She also learned long ago that rewarding herself for attaining her goals made working toward her goals a lot more fun.

The problem was that Sarah used food, specifically ice cream, as her primary reward for reaching short-term goals. It was cheap, pleasurable, and very abundant! As she aged and became more sedentary, the ice cream rewards began to add layers to her middle. When she realized that she had made food her primary reward for a job well done, she started using other rewards that would help her lose her excess weight.

Rewards that Sarah now uses include a healthy cooking magazine subscription, a pair of walking shoes, and a pedometer (step counter). She also decided to use free time as a reward. A full Saturday of reading romance novels, an evening on the phone with her former roommate, and a weekend trip with friends were great rewards. In fact, they had the added bonus of helping her reduce stress! ▮

? DID YOU KNOW?

Rewards Work

The Cooper Institute has conducted many studies on how people increase the amount of physical activity they get. They found that the people who increased their use of rewards were more likely to be doing the recommended amount of exercise three years later than people who did not increase their use of rewards. Do you want to change your eating habits? Try using rewards!

Food Monitoring

Now that you've set your goals and rewards, you need a way to see if you're on track to meet your goals. One way to measure whether you're moving in the right direction is to track your progress by self-monitoring. Self-monitoring, or recording what you eat, is one of the skills that has consistently been linked to success in changing eating habits. Keeping track of your food intake makes you more aware of what you're eating. Self-monitoring is especially important when you are just starting to make changes in your eating habits. By self-monitoring, you'll be able to see whether you really are making changes over time. Keeping a food log will also help you see opportunities to make changes as you're going through one day.

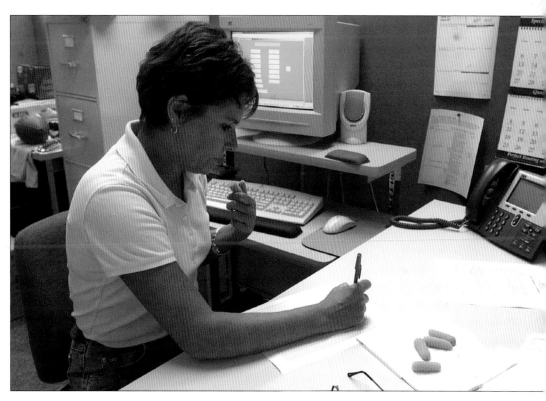

Use the Daily Food Log to monitor your eating habits.

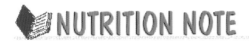

NUTRITION NOTE

Keeping Track

We'd like to introduce you to a form called the Daily Food Log that will help you develop the habit of self-monitoring. You'll notice that at the top of the form we ask you to identify a goal for the week. As you learned earlier in this session, goal setting is vital to your success in HEED. We suggest starting with the HEED goal area you identified earlier in this session as needing the most improvement, although you may choose another goal if you like. Try to limit yourself to one or two goals so that you can really focus on those areas. Next, in the area after the table in the form, fill in your recommended number of servings from each food group. This goes in the blank after "Total" in each row. Review table 1.2 (page 12) to refresh your memory about the number of servings you should be eating from each food group. Keep in mind that if you're inactive or trying to lose weight, you should choose a number on the low end of the range.

In the next column, you'll want to identify your goal servings for the day. This may not be the same as your recommended number of servings. For example, if you're focusing on increasing whole grains and you usually don't eat any servings of whole grains, your goal for the day may be to get one serving, not the recommended three. Because we want you to focus on one or two specific goals for the week, you may not have goal servings for all food groups. In other words, you can leave some blanks in the second column blank.

The next step is to record your daily food intake, using a process similar to the one you used for table 1.3 (page 14) in session 1 (see example on form). Simply write down everything you eat and drink during the day. For each item, record the amount you consumed, the food group it belongs to, and the number of food group servings the item amounts to. If your goal is to achieve caloric balance, you can use the last column to track the number of calories in each food. Look back to the guidelines in session 1 (page 11) if you need help judging serving sizes. Page 89 in session 7 and sessions 1 and 3 at HEED Online also provide examples of serving sizes. At the end of the day, total your food group servings and record them in the fourth column below the table, labeled "My servings today." Fill in one circle for each serving eaten. When you eat only one half of a serving, fill in one half of a circle.

Because the "Unsaturated fats and oils," "Saturated fats and trans fats," and "Sweets" categories do not have standard serving sizes, list the foods from these categories in the space provided. This will help you see what and how often you are eating these types of foods.

At the end of the form, identify whether you achieved your dietary improvement goals for the day. Feel free to write comments or reminders to yourself as to why you did or didn't achieve your goal. Remember, self-monitoring is exactly that: *self*-monitoring. Use this form to help you stay on track with the goals you have set for yourself.

Daily Food Log

Date: _____

My short-term healthy eating goals: _____

_____

_____

Meal	Food	Amount eaten	Food group (bread, fruits and vegetables, dairy, meat, fats, sweets)	Number of food group servings	Calories (optional)
Break-fast	Spinach omelet	3 eggs 1/4 cup (40 g) cooked spinach	Meat Fruits and veg-etables	1 1/2	220 10
	Orange juice	6 oz. (180 ml)	Fruits and veg-etables	1	82
	Nonfat milk	1 cup (240 ml)	Dairy	1	86
Lunch					
Dinner					
Snacks					

(continued)

(continued)

HEED pyramid food group		Recommended servings per day	My goal servings per day	My servings today ○ = 1 serving
Bread group	*Total*	_____	_____	○○○○○○○○○○○○
	Whole-grain (at least 3)		_____	○○○○○○
Fruit and vege-table group	*Total*	_____	_____	○○○○○○○○○○○
Dairy and dairy alterna-tives group	*Total*	_____	_____	○○○○○
	Low-fat or fat-free		_____	○○○○○
Meat and meat alterna-tives group	*Total*	_____	_____	○○○○○
	Lean meat, poultry, fish, legumes, nuts, and soy		_____	○○○○○

Unsaturated fats and oils (list here)

_____

Saturated fats and trans fats (list here)

_____

Sweets (list here)

_____

I attained my short-term healthy eating goals today (circle one): Yes   No

Comments _____

_____

Throughout HEED, we'll have reminders about self-monitoring and using the Daily Food Log to track your food intake. Make copies of the form from appendix B to use in the coming weeks. As you get more experience at food monitoring, you might find yourself keeping track of food servings in your head. That means you're becoming a self-monitoring pro! Until you get to that point, it's best to write down everything you eat immediately after you eat. This will help you see exactly what you're eating on a daily basis.

WEIGHTY MATTERS

This Meal Has *How* Many Calories?

You may think that counting calories is for the birds. But if your goal is to manage your weight, it's a necessary skill for you to develop. Here are some tips to help:

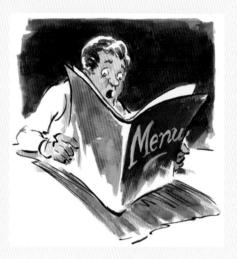

- Examine food labels for caloric content. Remember, calories listed are usually for *one serving* of the food.
- Scan menus for the healthy options. They will often have calories listed.
- Buy a book such that lists calories (and other nutrients) for foods and restaurant meals. You can find such a book at a local or online bookstore.

Session Checklist

Before you move on to the next session's activities, be sure to do the following:

- [ ] Complete the Ready? Set Goals! worksheet.

- [ ] Consider ideas for rewards that you would find motivating.

- [ ] Complete the Daily Food Log on a daily basis.

- [ ] Visit HEED Online for fun activities related to setting goals and rewards. You can also track your eating habits online.

You've done a lot in these first few sessions! With the completion of this session you now have the basic tools for healthy eating success. From sessions 1 and 2, you know what parts of your diet need help. In session 3, you set personal, realistic, specific, and measurable goals and rewards. You've learned how to monitor your food intake so that you know if you're on track. The next sessions will provide strategies and information that will help you reach your goals. We'll give you frequent opportunities to check your progress toward your goals. Each week you will set a weekly goal for change in one of the five HEED areas. Each week use the Daily Food Log to set a new weekly goal. You might already know of some barriers that are keeping you from reaching your goals. That's why in session 4 we'll look at the benefits of healthy eating. Then we'll take a hard look at how to overcome the barriers you might face in your quest to eat better.

FOUR

Identifying Barriers and Benefits

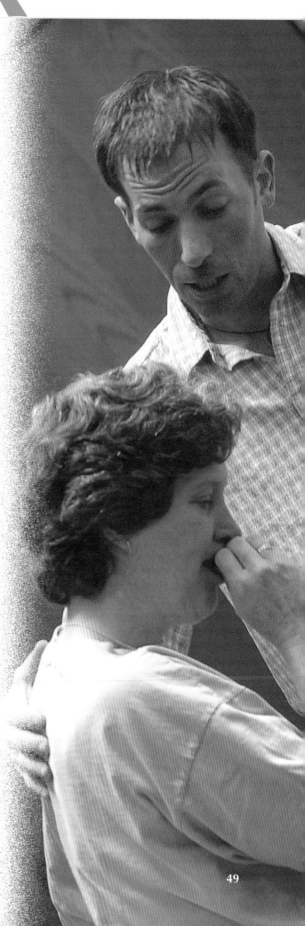

In This Session

- Identifying benefits of healthy eating
- Identifying barriers to healthy eating
- Problem solving to overcome barriers
- Increasing opportunities for healthy eating

Let's face it: Few people like to do anything without getting something in return. "What's in it for me?" we often ask. You're not likely to even try, much less stick with, new eating habits if you don't think you're going to benefit in some way. If you can think of a lot of barriers to changing your eating habits, chances are you're going to have to work more diligently to make new habits permanent. But don't be discouraged! In this session, you'll identify the benefits of changing your eating habits that are important to *you*. You'll also learn a creative method for problem solving your way through barriers, and you'll discover unexpected ways to eat better.

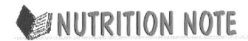

NUTRITION NOTE

Identifying My Benefits

If you find yourself asking, "What's in it for me?" you may be struggling to find a good reason for changing your eating habits. As with goal setting, it's important to have *personal* benefits that will motivate *you* to make changes. Let's look at some reasons why it's important to adopt healthier eating habits. In sessions 1 and 2, we shared some of the benefits we see for healthy eating, such as stronger bones, improved weight control, and a lower risk of certain cancers and heart disease. But these benefits might not matter to you. Read the questions below and think about the reasons you chose to pick up *Healthy Eating Every Day.*

How do you think you will benefit as you begin to eat in a healthier manner? What positive changes do you expect to see? List your answers in the space provided. Think of as many personal benefits as you can.

1. _____   6. _____

2. _____   7. _____

3. _____   8. _____

4. _____   9. _____

5. _____   10. _____

By answering these questions, you've identified your personal benefits of healthy eating.

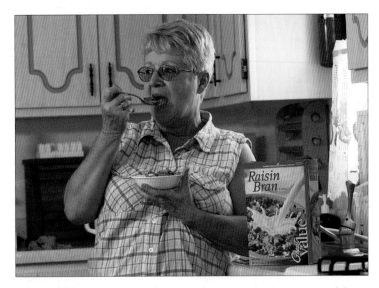

Eating whole-grain foods may reduce your risk of cancer and heart disease.

At this point, your list of benefits may be shorter than you expected. This is completely normal! In the weeks to come, you'll begin to see new benefits of healthy eating. If you had trouble listing benefits, here's some evidence from the scientific community that you might not have considered when generating your list. If you see any that are truly benefits to you, add them to your list.

- Eating a diet rich in whole grains, low-fat dairy products, fruits and vegetables, and lean meat, poultry, and fish can help people with high blood pressure reduce their blood pressure as much as some medications can.

- People who eat a fiber-rich diet with plenty of whole grains and fruits and vegetables are less likely to have coronary heart disease than are people who eat a diet with small amounts of fiber.

- Pregnant women who consume enough folic acid, which is found in certain whole grains, fruits, and vegetables, are less likely to have children with birth defects than are women who do not get enough folic acid.

- Men and women who eat dairy products and other calcium-rich foods are less likely than those who don't eat enough milk group foods to develop osteoporosis, a crippling bone disease that often leads to debilitating falls in older adults.

UP CLOSE AND PERSONAL

George decided he wanted to eat better. He had put on a lot of weight in the last 15 years. He had developed high cholesterol, and he was concerned that he might get diabetes later in life, like his mother had, if he didn't take better care of himself. Plus he simply wanted to feel better and have more energy. But George didn't really like "diet" food, and he traveled a lot. These factors had blocked him from successfully adopting better eating habits in the past.

George's brother, Patrick, also had high cholesterol and was overweight. In fact, Patrick's doctor had recently given him a stern warning about improving his diet. But Patrick loved to eat, and he figured he might as well die happy! Patrick worked odd hours, lived alone, ate out a lot, and didn't really know what a healthy diet was in the first place.

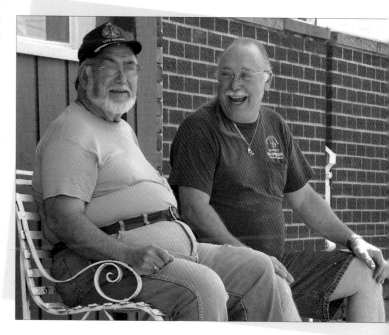

Who do you think was more successful at changing his diet? It was George. George could identify a lot more benefits of changing his diet than Patrick could. Also, although George had some major barriers to overcome, he didn't have as many as Patrick did. ▌

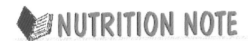

NUTRITION NOTE

Identifying My Barriers

What are the factors that keep you from eating a healthy diet? These can vary from environmental factors (such as co-workers who tempt you with sweets) to time management concerns to negative thoughts. A barrier is anything that could get in your way of making successful changes. Take some time to think about your barriers to healthy eating and list them here.

1. _____   6. _____

2. _____   7. _____

3. _____   8. _____

4. _____   9. _____

5. _____   10. _____

Don't be discouraged if you had a long list of barriers to healthy eating and fewer benefits. That's one of the reasons you're taking HEED—to get help in overcoming these barriers. Read on to find an IDEA for how to conquer the barriers that you've identified.

An IDEA for Busting Barriers

Identifying your personal barriers to healthy eating is an important first step in overcoming them. Now, how do you get past your healthy eating barriers? Developing your problem-solving skills can help you overcome the barriers that stand in your way.

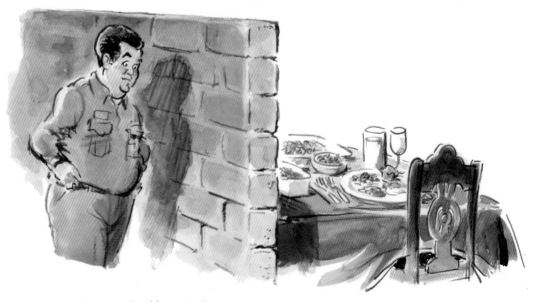

What are your barriers to healthy eating?

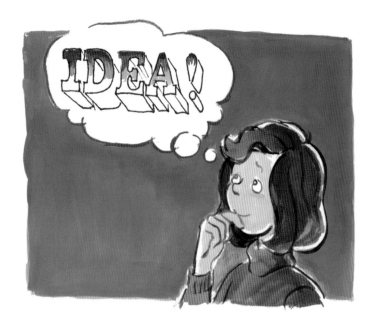

Problem solving involves creative thinking aimed at finding the most effective response to a situation. You can use many different methods to find solutions to problems. Here's one IDEA that you can use to overcome barriers. This strategy can be used to help you change many habits, not just your eating habits.

Identify the Problem

Choose one of your personal barriers and think through it thoroughly and specifically. For example, if family gatherings keep you from eating in a healthy manner, try to remember the events of the last family gathering. What specific thoughts and actions seemed to get in your way of eating healthy foods? Were you too busy to prepare healthy meals? Did you feel pressured to eat that extra piece of cake that your grandmother baked especially for you? The more specifically you can describe the problem, the more focused you can make the solution.

Develop a List of Possible Solutions

Think of as many possible solutions as you can. Do this by yourself or with a friend. Be creative. Don't limit yourself, and don't judge whether the solutions are good or bad. Try one of these approaches: Develop the longest list you can in 15 minutes or less, or think of all the ideas you can over a couple of days.

Evaluate Your Solutions

Now's the time to be realistic about your plan. Select one solution that you would be willing to try during the next week. Develop a specific plan to put your solution into practice. Remember, be as specific as you can. Describe how and when you are going to test your solution.

Analyze How Well Your Plan Worked

Periodically assess whether your plan is working. You might want to keep a copy of your plan on the refrigerator or by your desk at work. Your plan might not work the first time around. You may need to revise it by making a few minor changes or picking a different solution from the list you prepared. Other times you may need to start at the beginning of the IDEA process and redefine the problem.

People often skip the last step of the IDEA strategy and forget to analyze whether their solution really worked. Every step in the process is essential. It's as important to analyze and revise your plan as it is to identify the problem and develop solutions. It might take two or three tries before you choose the right solution for your barrier. Barriers will occur, but if you have developed problem-solving skills, you can handle any barrier that might come your way.

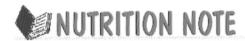 **NUTRITION NOTE**

Great IDEA!

Let's practice using the IDEA framework to help you overcome a barrier that you identified earlier in this session. This worksheet walks you through the IDEA strategy for problem solving. Use it to help you fine-tune your problem-solving skills.

I—Identify a barrier that keeps you from eating in a healthy manner.

_____

_____

_____

D—Develop a list of creative solutions. Accept every solution you think of as a possibility. Sometimes solutions you think won't work end up being the right ones.

_____

_____

_____

E—Evaluate the solutions. Select the solution you are most likely to implement. Then develop a specific plan to try it.

_____

_____

_____

A—After implementing the plan, analyze how well it worked. Do you need to make any changes? Revise your plan if you need to. Write down dates on your calendar when you will review your plan again.

_____

_____

_____

Once you've identified your barrier, listed possible solutions, and selected the solution you'll try, you're ready to implement the plan during the coming week. Follow your plan for the next week. At the end of the week, analyze your plan to see if it worked. If it didn't work, revise your plan and try again. You probably won't change your habits overnight, but if you keep trying, over time you'll start to notice successful changes.

UP CLOSE AND PERSONAL

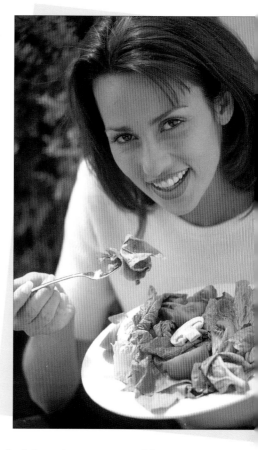

Nicole is a 29-year-old mother of two children ages 7 and 5. She works in the accounting department for a medium-sized company. Her husband, Don, teaches at the local school. Nicole was raised in a "meat and potatoes" household in which fruits and vegetables were rarely served. This pattern has carried over into her own household. Today, Nicole knows that she and her family should eat more fruits and vegetables. She'd like to get the health benefits they offer and set a good example for her kids. Nicole wants to increase her daily intake of fruits and vegetables to the five to nine servings that are right for her.

The first step for Nicole was to **identify** her specific barriers to eating more fruits and vegetables. She recognized that her two biggest barriers were that (1) it was hard to find fruits and vegetables on a menu when eating out, and (2) she didn't think she or her children liked the taste of many vegetables. Nicole decided to focus on the second barrier first.

Nicole asked her husband to help her **develop** possible solutions to her barriers. They spent a few minutes writing down all the possible ways they could think of to make vegetables more appealing. They came up with ideas such as stir-frying vegetables, trying new vegetable recipes, using low-fat salad dressing on vegetables, doubling the amount of vegetables eaten at mealtimes, and many others. They laughed about some of the unhealthy ideas they thought of, such as smothering vegetables in cheese or butter!

After **evaluating** which ideas were acceptable, Nicole and Don decided to try new recipes. Because Nicole hadn't been exposed to many vegetables as a kid, she was willing to try some new ones. They went to a produce Web site for ideas. Together they chose a handful of recipes that they could try during the coming week.

After a week, Nicole **assessed** her plan by reviewing her daily food logs to see how many vegetable servings she was eating. With the new recipes in hand and with Don's help, she averaged about three servings of vegetables per day. Along with the fruits she was already eating, she was getting a lot closer to the recommended level than she had been. Plus, the entire family had discovered some new vegetables that they enjoyed. Nicole didn't stop there. Next, she decided to simply double up on her vegetable serving size, while reducing her meat portion. Soon she was getting the five to nine servings of fruits and vegetables that she needs each day, and her children were eating much better, too.

Nicole not only successfully implemented the IDEA strategy, but she also used other skills to help overcome her barrier. Nicole monitored her progress by using her daily food log. This helped her see whether she was meeting her goal. Nicole also sought support from her husband by involving him in the process. You'll learn more about enlisting social support in session 9. ∎

Finding Healthy Opportunities

The environment that you live in might be a barrier to healthy eating. Your surroundings are constantly changing, and often for the worse when it comes to healthy eating. For example, think about how restaurant portion sizes have grown in recent decades. You can even get giant-sized drinks at most fast food restaurants and convenience stores. In many countries, it's unlikely that we'll return to a time when families spent hours cooking homemade, nutritious meals, and eating out was considered a special occasion. Because of our changing environment, you might feel as if the whole world is against you in your attempts to improve your eating habits.

But for every ad, sign, fast food restaurant, or corner convenience store, there are plenty of healthy food options waiting for you to explore. You may have to broaden your horizons to find all the healthy opportunities available. Even fast food restaurants and convenience stores offer healthy choices. You'll learn more about choosing healthy options when eating away from home in session 6, and we'll discuss more about our changing food environment in session 18. For now, let's think about some different resources where you can find out more about healthy eating. This can include Web sites with nutrition information, magazines with healthy recipes, or vendors in your area who sell fresh produce or healthy meals–to go. See if any of these resources interest you:

Web Sites

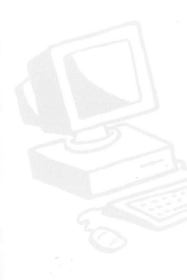

American Dietetic Association (www.eatright.org). This site has many tips and ideas for consumers who want to eat healthier. Be sure to go to "Healthy Lifestyle Tips" under "Food and Nutrition Information."

American Heart Association (www.americanheart.org). This general information site is full of information about diet and heart disease. For more specific information about food and nutrition from the American Heart Association go to www.deliciousdecisions.org.

Dietitians of Canada (www.dietitians.ca). This Web site brings you up-to-date information about dietetic research, while also providing a variety of resources to help readers make healthy food choices and learn more about nutrition.

Books, Newsletters, and Magazines

Stealth Health: How to Sneak Nutrition Painlessly into Your Diet by Evelyn Tribole (Penguin USA, 2000).

The Complete Book of Food Counts, 6th edition, by Corinne T. Netzer (Dell, 2003).

Tufts University Health & Nutrition Letter

Subscription Department

P.O. Box 420235

Palm Coast, FL 32142-0235

800-274-7581

Cooking Light magazine

www.cookinglight.com/cooking/magazine

Vendors

Local farmers' markets—You'll get fresh produce and support your local growers.

Specialty grocery stores—Many cities have grocery stores that specialize in organic foods or various ethnic cuisines. You can get information from them on preparing healthy foods from different regions of the world.

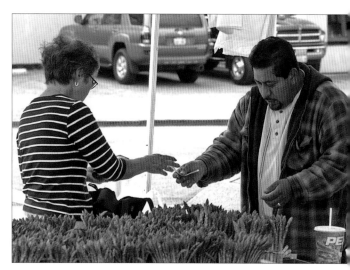

You can get fresh produce at farmers' markets.

Cooking classes—Some grocery stores and professional cooking schools offer cooking lessons for amateur cooks who are eager to learn the "tricks of the trade." Check with your local stores and schools for schedules and prices.

NUTRITION NOTE

Opportunities for Healthy Eating

We hope this list has given you a few ideas that will help you identify healthy opportunities in your local area. Now it's your turn! Using the worksheet Opportunities for Healthy Eating, try to list at least 10 things you could do to learn more about healthy eating or to practice healthy eating in new ways. If you have trouble thinking of ideas on your own, recruit a friend or family member to help you. Choose one idea that you can put into action this week.

Think of ways to learn more about healthy eating or *new* ways you can practice healthy eating. Come up with as long a list as possible and *be creative!*

Ways to learn more about healthy eating	New ways to practice healthy eating
Search on "whole-grain recipes" on the Internet	*Add one serving of fruit to my lunch*

(continued)

(continued)

_____   _____

_____   _____

_____   _____

_____   _____

_____   _____

_____   _____

You can use this list when you're thinking of ways to overcome your barriers. When developing your IDEA plan for problem solving, see if any of the ideas you wrote on this list will lead to a solution. You might also want to look at appendix C, which includes even more tips pertaining to the five HEED goal areas.

Session Checklist

Before you move on to the next session's activities, be sure to do the following:

- ☐ Complete the Great IDEA! worksheet and implement your solution.

- ☐ Complete the Opportunities for Healthy Eating worksheet.

- ☐ Complete the Daily Food Log on a daily basis.

- ☐ Visit HEED Online for more ideas on healthy eating away from home.

In this session you listed your benefits and barriers to healthy eating, you learned the IDEA strategy for problem solving, and you thought of ways to find opportunities for healthy eating in your environment. You've probably found that certain events or situations make you want to eat in unhealthy ways. Perhaps you eat unhealthy food when under stress. Or maybe struggle to fit in healthy food when your schedule becomes busy. In session 5, we'll help you find ways to control these eating triggers.

FIVE

Tackling Triggers

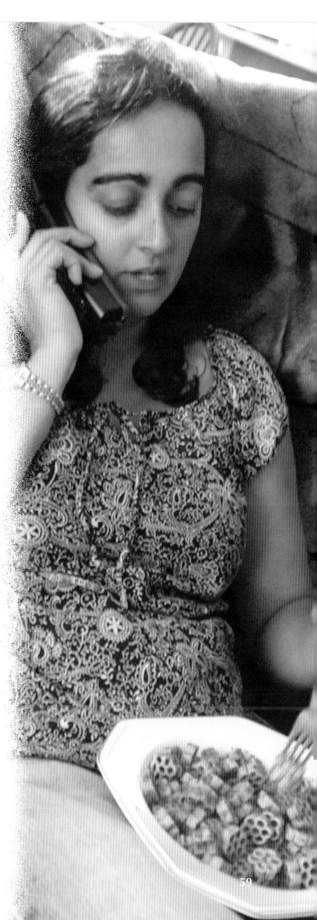

In This Session

- Defining hunger
- Identifying and dealing with eating triggers
- Understanding nutrient density

Most living creatures are driven to eat by hunger. But for us humans, many other things besides hunger affect our eating habits. In fact, our world is filled with all kinds of *triggers* for unhealthy eating. This session will explore how you can become more aware of the things that may lead you to eat a poor diet.

The Hunger Dilemma

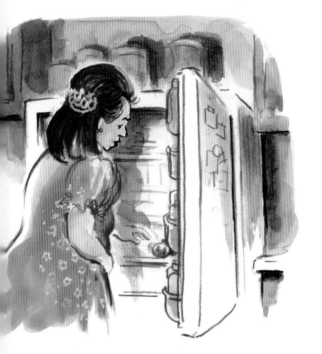

Sadly, for many people around the world, hunger is a daily companion. Such **physiological hunger** has physical symptoms such as an empty feeling in the stomach, headaches, or lightheadedness. You may have felt some of these symptoms when you skipped a meal or two. They are signs that your body needs more fuel in the form of calories and nutrients. When you feel physiological hunger, you need to eat.

But many people living in countries in which food is plentiful and inexpensive experience another type of hunger. Thoughts of food even soon after a meal, cravings, or particular triggers for eating are examples of **psychological hunger.** Psychological hunger occurs when there are no physical indicators that it is time to refuel your body. You just feel as if you want to eat something. Psychological hunger is usually caused by an environmental or internal trigger. Such triggers might include smelling food (hot pie fresh from the oven), social situations, or your mood. Eating because of psychological hunger can lead to eating too many calories and unhealthy foods. Let's look at triggers in more detail.

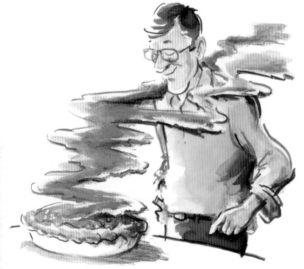

Internal and External Triggers

We are faced with many different eating triggers every day. Many are *external*—they come from your environment. Your *internal* thoughts and mood can also act as eating triggers. And as we learned earlier, needing to refuel the body can be another eating trigger. Circle the triggers for eating that you find in Robert's story:

🔍 UP CLOSE AND PERSONAL

Once a month, Robert's family gathers for a big family meal around 4:00 p.m. Because he knew he was going to have a big meal, Robert decided to skip breakfast and had only a piece of fruit for lunch. When he walked in the door of his sister's house and saw all the familiar foods and smelled all the wonderful aromas, he was overcome with anxiety. *How am I ever going to stick with my eating goals?* he asked himself. But quickly Robert stopped his thoughts: *This is my day off. I just need to relax, have fun, and forget about trying to eat in a healthy way for one day.* Robert sat down in the living room with his relatives and ate several large chunks of cheese since he was very hungry. He didn't really like this appetizer, but he was quite hungry.

Robert felt full before he even sat down at the table. Still, when dinner was served, he enjoyed the large meal and ate everything from the bread to the potatoes. He felt really full halfway through the meal but felt obliged to clean his plate. Dessert came next and he told himself that he would eat a little so that he wouldn't offend his grandmother. But the chocolate cake was just too good to stop at a small piece. Finally the meal ended, and Robert felt like he

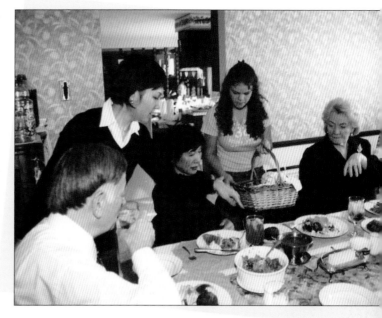

was about to burst. His family stayed around the table for a couple hours talking and telling stories. Robert enjoyed the time with his family, but he felt bored after the first 30 minutes. Restless, he unconsciously reached for some sweets to keep him occupied. Robert left his sister's home later that evening feeling overly full and frustrated, promising himself that the next Sunday would be different. ▮

This is probably a familiar story for a lot of people. How many triggers did you find? We count eight separate things that influenced Robert's eating: physical hunger, anxiety about not meeting his healthy eating goals, seeing foods, smelling foods, feeling obligated to clean his plate, not wanting to offend his grandmother, the great taste of the chocolate cake, and boredom.

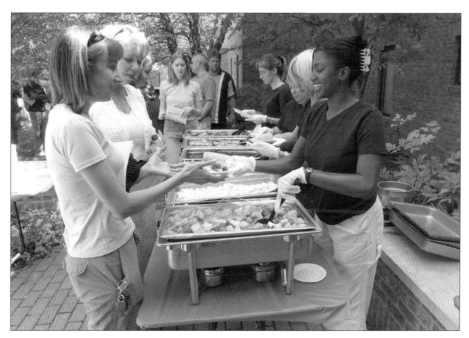

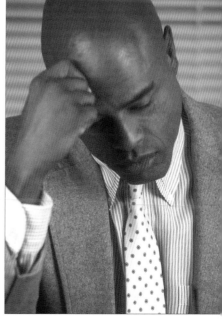

Are you more influenced by external triggers, such as food at a party, or internal triggers, such as certain emotions?

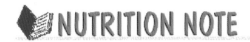

Identifying My Eating Triggers

Every person is different. It's important to learn if psychological triggers are problems for you and, if so, how you can combat them. In the form provided, mark the eating triggers that are problems for you. If you are aware of other personal eating triggers, list them in the space provided.

External triggers
I tend to eat when I am not hungry when I . . .

❏   see food
❏   smell food
❏   drink alcohol
❏   am at work or business functions
❏   am at parties or social functions
❏   am on vacation or holiday
❏   am with certain people
❏   read
❏   watch TV
❏   cook
❏   talk on the phone

Internal triggers
I tend to eat when I am not hungry when I feel . . .

❏   happy
❏   tired
❏   bored
❏   sad
❏   upset or angry
❏   anxious
❏   disappointed or hurt
❏   overloaded

Other external or internal triggers:

_____
_____
_____
_____
_____
_____
_____
_____
_____

I tend to eat when I am not hungry . . .
❏   before breakfast
❏   before lunch
❏   before dinner
❏   after dinner
❏   in the middle of the night

Coping With Triggers

Just about everyone has a few cues that trigger inappropriate eating. Eating a healthier diet depends, in part, on knowing how to respond to these triggers. When you feel the urge to eat, you need to determine if what you feel is physiological (physical) hunger or psychological hunger. If it is physical hunger, then you need to eat something, hopefully something healthy and in a proper portion size! If you want to eat something but you're not physically hungry, then you need to find out what is triggering you to eat. Once you have determined the trigger, you can decide whether to *adapt* to or *avoid* the trigger.

Adapt—Sometimes the best way to break the association between specific triggers and unhealthy eating is to replace the triggers with a different activity or to change your situation. For example, say you work out of your car most of the time because you are usually on the road visiting clients. You tend to often eat at fast food restaurants because they are quick and inexpensive. So eating out and needing to eat quickly are triggers for unhealthy eating. Obviously you can't give up your job, but you can adapt these triggers. You could pack a lunch and keep it in a cooler in your car. You could also go to fast food restaurants that offer healthy choices.

Be careful. During the times when you are struggling with a trigger, you may not be able to readily think of alternative activities. It's helpful to think of strategies ahead of time so that you have alternatives in place when a trigger occurs.

Avoid—If you have worked hard to adapt to certain situations and you still eat inappropriately, you may need to try ways to avoid those situations. For example, you might find that you tend to eat when you are bored. You will need to identify when those times seem to occur (at night, on weekends, during holidays) and then plan alternative activities that will help keep you from eating inappropriately.

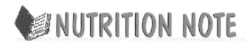

NUTRITION NOTE

Tackling My Triggers

Now it's your turn to tackle a couple of your own triggers. Select two of the eating triggers you identified in the chart on page 62. Choose one trigger to adapt to and one trigger to avoid. Think about the strategies you can use to adapt to one of the triggers. List your ideas in the space provided. For the other trigger, think of ways you can avoid it altogether.

Adapt

Trigger: _____

Ways to adapt your situation: _____

_____

_____

_____

Avoid

Trigger: _____

Ways to avoid your situation: _____

_____

_____

_____

Here are a few more tips for tackling triggers:

- Think about how your stomach, mouth, and head feel. If you don't feel physical symptoms of hunger, try to figure out what is prompting you to want to eat. Maybe you are just thirsty.
- Eat slowly. It takes a while for your brain to receive the signal from your stomach that you are full. If you eat fast, you can easily overeat before the signal gets through to your brain.
- Pause in the middle of a meal or snack to do a fullness check. If you are no longer hungry, stop eating. Save what is left on your plate for another meal.
- Once you feel that you have had enough, reinforce your conscious decision to stop. For example, nudge your plate forward, or put your utensils or napkin on your plate.
- Eat without distraction. Try to eat in the same place or at least sit down when eating so that you can enjoy the food. Don't do other things such as read or watch television.

Dense Diets

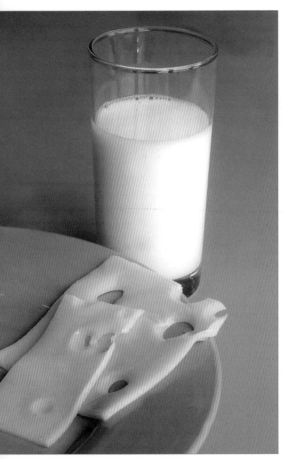

As you have seen, eating is often influenced by external triggers in our everyday world (such as sights, sounds, and smells) and by internal triggers (such as mood, feelings, and fatigue). Attitudes and beliefs about food can also influence what we eat. Many people believe that foods such as sweets, chips, and pizza are junk food and off limits in a healthy diet. But studies show that people who excessively restrict their favorite foods often end up overindulging in them. It seems that a negative attitude about these foods can cause a lot of guilt and remorse when they are eaten. These bad feelings can trigger unhealthy eating.

So in HEED, there are no "good" foods or "bad" foods. We know that to make and maintain healthy changes in your diet, the changes have to be something that you can live with—for a lifetime! In other words, *all* foods can fit.

Even though we think there is no such thing as "bad" or "junk" foods, some foods are definitely more nutritious than others. Considering *nutrient density* is one way to help you make healthier choices. Nutrient density is a measure of the nutrients in a food relative to the energy (calories) it provides. The more nutrients a food has and the fewer the calories, the higher the nutrient density of that food. For example, 1-1/2 ounces (45 g) of Swiss cheese, similar to Emmental cheese, and 8 ounces (240

Compare nutrient density: 1-1/2 ounces (45 g) of Swiss cheese, similar to Emmental cheese, has 132 calories. One cup (240 ml) of nonfat milk has only 80 calories. Both provide the same amount of calcium.

ml) of nonfat milk both contain about 300 milligrams of calcium. But the cheese has nearly twice as many calories as the milk because it has more fat. Therefore, the nonfat milk is more nutrient dense than the cheese. This makes the milk a more nutritious choice.

Table 5.1 provides some more specific guidance in determining the nutrient density of the foods you eat. For each food group, the foods that are more nutrient rich are listed toward the top of the table. Foods that have a lot of calories and few or no nutrients are listed toward the bottom. Again, we are not saying that you should never eat the foods that are at the bottom of the table. However, such low-nutrient-dense foods should be eaten in moderation—in small quantities and infrequently.

Table 5.1 Nutrient Density by Food Group

	Bread group	Fruit and vegetable group	Dairy and dairy alternatives	Meat and meat alternatives	Fats and oils	Sweets
High nutrient density	Whole-grain or bran cereal	Spinach	Nonfat milk	Fish	Canola oil	
		Cantaloupe (rockmelon)				
			Plain yogurt	Legumes		
	Whole-wheat bread	Broccoli			Olive oil	
	Oatmeal	Berries	1% milk	Soy products		
		Mango				
		Cauliflower		Poultry	Liquid margarine	
		Oranges	2% milk			
	Potatoes	Red and green peppers				
				Lean meats and game meats	Tub (soft) margarine	
	Sweet corn	Watermelon	Low-fat cheese			
		Tomatoes				
		Carrots				
	White bread	Apples	Sweetened yogurt	Nuts		
		100% fruit juice			Stick (hard) margarine	Chocolates
	Sweetened cereal	Dried fruit		Eggs		Cakes
		Cabbage	Chocolate milk	Fatty meats	Butter	Cookies (biscuits in Australia and the UK)
	Doughnuts	Green beans		Sausage, bacon		
	French fries (chips in the UK)	Celery	Whole milk	Fried meats, poultry, and fish	Shortening	Pies
		Sweetened fruit juice			Lard	Honey
	Potato chips (crisps in the UK)	Iceberg lettuce	Regular cheese			Jam
		Chocolate-covered raisins			Drippings, in the UK	Licorice
Low nutrient density						Sweetened beverages

As you look at table 5.1, circle the foods you regularly eat in each food category. Are most of your choices closer to the bottom or the top of each list? Remember that there are no "bad" foods. You shouldn't overly restrict your favorite foods: Doing so may lead you to binge on them at some point. But most of your diet should come from foods that are more nutrient dense. In fact, some dietitians recommend living by the 80/20 rule, in which 80% of the foods you consume are nutrient dense and healthy, and the other 20% are from the less nutrient-dense options. Any progress toward a healthier way of eating is important. If your diet is currently 20/80, improving to even 50/50 will help you reap extensive benefits!

Becoming a healthy eater takes time and practice. You don't have to be perfect 100% of the time. Eating should be a pleasurable experience, so enjoy your food. If you want a rich dessert, don't deny yourself. Just have a smaller portion or share it with a friend. It is your overall diet that counts, not just one meal. And enjoy all aspects of food—taste, texture, aroma, and appearance. Remember, what counts is that you make gradual progress toward your goals.

Session Checklist

Before you move on to the next session's activities, be sure to do the following:

- ◼ Complete the Identifying My Eating Triggers worksheet.

- ◼ Complete the Tackling My Triggers worksheet.

- ◼ Complete the Daily Food Log on a daily basis.

- ◼ Visit HEED Online for more activities about triggers and learning how "all foods can fit."

Unlike many countries around the world, most Western nations have a great abundance of food. We are bombarded with messages to eat all day long. Paying attention to and controlling eating triggers is one way to minimize less healthy foods and to maximize the nutrient content of the foods you eat. Understanding that all foods can fit into a healthy diet is another very important part of the journey toward healthy eating. The next session will help you learn specific strategies for healthy eating when eating out.

SIX

Eating Out

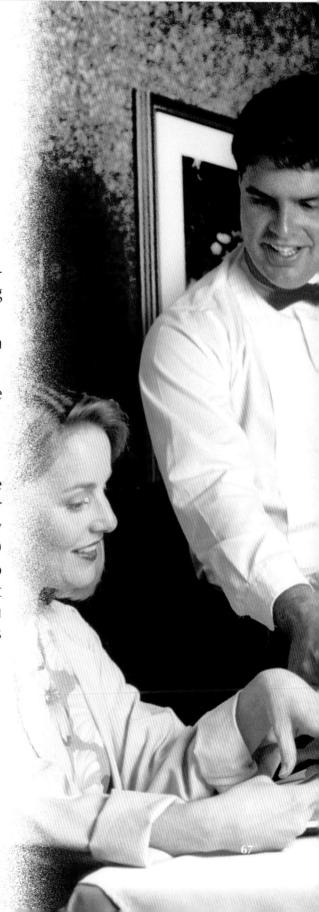

In This Session

- Knowing the difference between necessity eating out and special occasion eating out

- Learning the skill of defensive dining when eating out

- Developing strategies for eating on the run

We know that for most people, eating out is here to stay. But is it possible for you to maintain your busy lifestyle, eat out often, and still eat a healthy diet? The answer is yes. One of the goals of HEED is to help you make healthier dietary choices no matter where you eat. Whether you eat at a fast food establishment or a sit-down restaurant, you will need to use some defensive dining strategies to stick with your healthy eating goals.

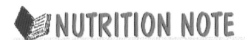
DID YOU KNOW?

The trends in eating out are astounding! In the United States in 2000, 76% of all Americans reported eating at least one commercially prepared meal each week. Not only are we more likely to eat out each week, but the frequency of eating out has also increased. In 2000, Americans were 40% more likely to eat out three or more times each week than they were in 1987.[12] We're also spending more of our food budget on food away from home (figure 6.1). Unfortunately, U.S.

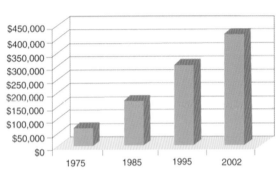

Figure 6.1 Total expenditures (in millions of U.S. dollars) on food away from home.

surveys show that meals that are eaten away home have more total and saturated fat than is present in foods that are eaten at home. The trends are similar in many Western countries, though the United Kingdom is an exception. This does not mean that we can't get healthy foods at restaurants. But it does mean that it may take a little more work and practice to make healthier choices when eating out.

NUTRITION NOTE

Defensive Dining

If you are like most people, you have probably noticed that you eat away from home more than you used to. You also may have noticed that the foods you eat away from home are not as nutritious as the foods you eat at home. To help you identify what strategies can best help you stay on track with your healthy eating goals, take this quiz.

For the questions below, "eating out" refers to any time you acquire and eat any food away from your home. Don't count foods that you prepare at home and eat elsewhere (such as food you take on picnics, in lunches, or to parties). Select either "a" or "b" for each item.

Question 1
  a. On average I eat out two times or less per week.
  b. On average I eat out three or more times per week.

Question 2
  a. I usually eat out just for special occasions.
  b. I usually eat out for everyday meals or snacks.

Question 3
  a. I eat mostly at restaurants where I sit down and order off a menu.
  b. I eat mostly at places where I can get the food quickly and leave.

Question 4

    a. I don't mind paying a little more for a good meal.

    b. I want food that tastes good but is not expensive.

Question 5

    a. I am willing to travel across town to get a meal.

    b. I want to go to restaurants and convenience stores that are easy to get to.

Question 6

    a. I spend at least an hour or two when eating out.

    b. I spend 10 to 30 minutes when eating out.

Question 7

    a. I live in an area that has few restaurant choices.

    b. I live in an area that has many restaurants.

Add together the number of "a" options you selected: _____

Add together the number of "b" options you selected: _____

If the total of your "a" choices is greater than that of your "b" choices, you are a *special occasion diner*. But if you chose "b" more often than "a," you are a *necessity diner*.

So what? Knowing your eating-out style will help you decide how to best improve your eating habits when eating away from home. If you are a special occasion diner, you don't have to be as vigilant as a necessity diner when eating out. As a special occasion diner, you eat out less frequently and have more options available to you when you eat out. You tend to eat more slowly, you can easily make special requests, and you rarely have to contend with pressures and promotions to supersize your meal. Now don't get carried away. If you're a special occasion diner, you still have to be mindful of your choices, but you have a little more leeway than do people who eat away from home out of necessity.

Don't despair if you are a necessity diner. Most of us are. However, if you're a necessity diner you are at greater risk of eating unhealthy foods when eating

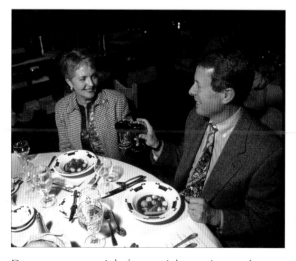 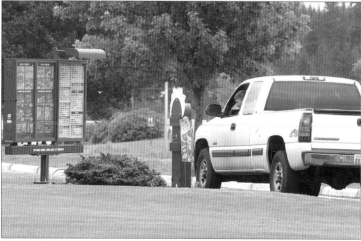

Do you eat out mainly for special occasions or for many everyday meals? Either way, HEED can help.

out than are special occasion diners. Why? Because you often eat out at places that have limited menus and service, offer little in the way of healthy side dishes, and push the extra-large "value" deals that pile on the calories and fat. Read on to learn defensive dining strategies for both the special occasion diner (see below through page 72) and the necessity diner (see pages 72 to 76). The following tips are keys to success no matter what your style.

Planning Leads to Success

One way to ensure that you're prepared to make the right food choices is to plan ahead. Ask yourself these questions to help you start thinking about healthy ways to eat out:

What restaurants or food sources offer healthy options?

Ask friends if they know of restaurants that offer healthy options. Try new places yourself. Many restaurants post their menus on the Internet, and some even provide nutrition information about their menu items online.

What healthy options are available at each place?

One restaurant might simply have a salad bar as one part of a wide-ranging and not-so-healthy menu. But another restaurant might be entirely devoted to healthy foods. The more healthy options a menu includes, the more likely you are to find one that will agree with your taste buds and your healthy eating goals.

What will I choose when I get there?

Before you walk into a food establishment, decide what you are going to choose. You don't have to know the exact item. But try to have a general idea, such as, "I'm going to order a salad and grilled fish and share a dessert." Or, "I am going to buy a bottle of tomato juice and a small bag of peanuts." If you wait until you get inside, you may be tempted by menu items or store displays that are not the healthiest options.

❓ DID YOU KNOW?

Two tablespoons of regular salad dressing can have as much as 18 grams of fat. Keep this in mind the next time you "do the right thing" and order a salad. Look for reduced-fat salad dressings or limit the amount of regular dressing that you use.

Special Occasion Dining Strategies

If you are a special occasion diner, these tips will steer you toward healthy choices. If you're a necessity diner, think about how you can use these tips when you dine out.

Mind the Menu

Even the most health-conscious consumers can have problems deciding what the healthy options are on restaurant menus. Here are some tips that you can use to be a smart customer:

- Watch out for entrees that are described as au gratin, crispy, creamy, cheesy, breaded, battered, scalloped, sauteed, or fried. They are typically high in calories and fat. Instead, look for steamed, poached, baked, braised, broiled, or grilled.
- Maximize your nutrition by choosing dark green leafy greens (such as spinach or romaine) over light green lettuce (such as iceberg).
- Choose broth-based soups. Minestrone soup often includes a lot of vegetables. Lentil or dried bean soup can be good options, too, if they are not thickened with cream or cheese.
- Look for tomato-based instead of cream- or cheese-based sauces when ordering pasta or Mexican food.
- Broiled, baked, and grilled poultry or meats can be good entree choices. For lower-calorie options choose poultry without the skin, veal, fish, or lean cuts of beef such as filet mignon, top sirloin, flank, top round steak or top round roast (often called London broil in the U.S.), or shish kebob.
- You can increase the nutrient content of your meal by choosing a vegetable dish, vegetable soup, double portions of vegetable side dishes (as long as they are not smothered in cheese or cream sauce), an order of sliced tomatoes, or fresh fruit to complement your entree.
- Order fresh fruit or sorbet for dessert. If a richer dessert looks irresistible, share it with a friend.

Cut Your Portions Down to Size

Many restaurants know that customers want value, so they serve large portions. Remember the HEED pyramid serving guidelines from session 1? Most portions served at restaurants count as two to three servings!

- Ask for a bag or box to take half your meal home. You won't be as likely to overeat, and you'll have a meal to take home for another day.

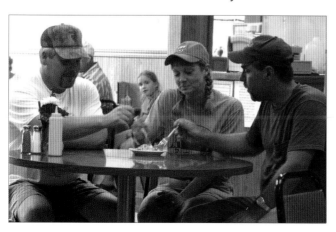

If you're tempted to have dessert, reduce your portion size by sharing it with a friend.

- Ask your server to put half of your meal in a take-home container before bringing out your meal. That way you won't be tempted to eat the complete meal all at one time.
- Share a meal with a friend. You can each order your own salads and then split the entree. Order extra sides of steamed vegetables to help fill you up. It's more economical and better for you.
- Request a half-portion of an entree.
- Share one dessert among several people.
- Order the a la carte, child, or lunch portion even at dinner meals.

Have It Your Way

Don't feel limited by the selections or the preparation methods that are listed on the menu. Most restaurants will make modifications to recipes and menu items upon request. Remember—you are paying for your meal and you deserve to get exactly what you want! To order with confidence, ask the server

- to describe menu items that you are not sure about;
- if they have a menu that lists the nutritional values of items;
- if they have low-fat or low-calorie choices;
- to substitute a small salad, fresh vegetables, or fruit for high-fat items such as french fries or chips; and
- to put sauces, butter, or dressings on the side or to omit them altogether.

Other Special Occasion Tips

See if any of these additional tips will help you as you strive to reach your goals even as you eat out.

- To save calories, decide to have either an appetizer or a dessert, but not both.
- To save calories, limit alcohol. Also, too much alcohol can reduce your resolve to make healthy choices.
- Be the first to order so that you are not swayed by what other people order.
- Slow your eating by trying to keep pace with the slowest eater at the table.
- Pass the bread or chips basket to the opposite side of the table.
- Don't skip meals if you are planning to eat out later. Instead, perhaps eat a little less. Completely skipping a meal will cause you to be overly hungry when you arrive for your meal out. That can quickly lead to overeating.
- Take time to savor the flavors of your meal and enjoy the company of family, friends, or colleagues.

Eating in the Melting Pot

Ethnic cuisines are the fastest-growing segment of the restaurant industry. People are looking for new flavors, and the shrinking of the globe is making it easy for us to try exotic and not-so-exotic foods. Some imported menu items are better choices than others. Go to session six of HEED Online at www.ActiveLiving.info for a list of recommended foods for many different ethnic cuisines.

Necessity Dining Strategies

As the label implies, necessity diners eat out because they perceive that they have to eat out in order to eat at all. Many of us can relate! You might be a necessity diner because you don't like to cook or you don't feel comfortable in the kitchen. Or it could be that you don't have time to go food shopping and prepare meals at home. The convenience and perceived value of foods from quick-service restaurants or convenience stores make it easy to simply pick up something on the way to or from work, the kids' sports practice, appointments, or community events.

? DID YOU KNOW?

A recent study conducted in Minnesota measured the frequency of fast food restaurant use among adolescents. The researchers found that students who more frequently ate at fast food restaurants consumed more total calories, more calories from fat, and fewer servings of fruit, vegetables, and milk than did students who ate at fast food restaurants less frequently.[13]

If you're a necessity diner, one of the best strategies for improving your diet is to reduce the number of times per week that you eat out. This is possible if you do the following:

- Prepare more of your food at home. In session 12, we'll talk about simple and fast healthy cooking strategies such as using a Crock-Pot and cooking with frozen food. We'll also show you a faster way of making meals from scratch. You might want to check out the dozens of cookbooks, Web sites, and magazines that offer tips for making healthy food fast.

- Prepare healthy food at home to take with you for breakfast, lunch to eat at your desk, or healthy snacks to eat between meetings. If you have to eat out, bring your own piece of fruit or fresh vegetables to add to your meal.

- Involve your family members. They can learn valuable healthy cooking techniques and make meal preparation go faster. As an added bonus, you'll spend more time together, something that many families yearn for.

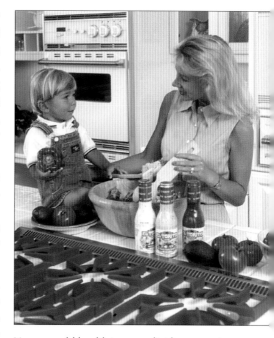

You can add health to your diet by preparing more food at home.

Even if you are successful at reducing the number of meals you eat out each week, you'll probably still eat out occasionally. Let's look at various quick-service food outlets and the healthy options that they offer.

Fast Food Restaurants

Fast food establishments have become a staple of Western economies for many reasons:

- They offer a kid- and family-friendly environment.
- They are relatively inexpensive.
- The food is familiar.

- Eating their meals is fast and easy.
- They are conveniently located.
- They offer numerous options for picky eaters.
- There are more dual income households now than ever before, leaving less time for home cooking and leading more families to look for quick and inexpensive ways to eat.

However, the fast food industry has become the target of criticism from nutrition and health care professions for several reasons:

- Obesity rates have increased with the proliferation of fast food chains.
- Childhood diabetes rates are increasing faster than ever before.
- Serving sizes have grown to more than two or three times their original size.
- Marketing campaigns by the fast food industry are aimed at influencing the choices of young children and teenagers.
- Fast food choices are now available in many school cafeterias.

All finger-pointing aside, you are in charge of the food that goes into your body. No matter how much we would like to blame the fast food industry for force-feeding a double cheeseburger down our throats, we must learn to make better choices when we have to eat at fast food restaurants and other convenient eating locations. Thanks to consumer demand and industry concern over the battle with the bulge, more healthy options are available than ever before. Next time you eat at a fast food restaurant, consider one of these options:

- Meal-sized and side salads (Ask for the fat-free or light dressing or use very little of the regular dressing. A full packet of regular dressing can add over 400 calories and a lot of fat to a low-fat salad.)
- Regular hamburgers
- Vegetarian hamburgers
- Small roast beef sandwiches
- Grilled chicken sandwiches on buns or rolls (In the U.S., avoid sandwiches with biscuits or croissants.)
- Soft chicken or bean tacos
- Deli or submarine sandwiches without mayonnaise or special sauces
- Baked potatoes (top with chili; use little or no cheese)
- Pancakes
- Fruit and yogurt options
- Fat-free muffins
- Egg on English muffins or bagels*
- Low-fat milk
- 100% juice
- Water
- Diet soft drinks

*In the United States, skip the croissant or biscuit version.

Remember, it's easier to start with a healthier option such as a grilled chicken sandwich and leave off the mayonnaise than it is to start with a triple cheeseburger and try to make it into a healthy option. Here are some easy strategies for improving fast food meals:

- Get out of your burger, fries, and soft drink rut. Be daring and try a salad, grilled chicken sandwich, or yogurt and fruit.
- Leave out high-fat condiments such as mayonnaise, tartar sauce, butter, or margarine.
- Reduce the amount of regular cheese, sour cream, guacamole, salad dressing, and olives that you use.
- Add more vegetables than usual to a hamburger or sandwich.
- Use a reduced-fat salad dressing in place of regular salad dressing. Eat a baked potato or mashed potatoes instead of french fries.*
- Avoid supersizing meals unless you are sharing them.

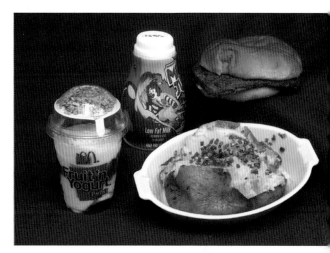

Healthier options from fast food restaurants: regular hamburger, baked potato with few toppings, low-fat milk, and a fruit and yogurt dessert.

Convenience Stores

You'll probably find yourself eating on the run at one time or another. As you know, it's not just fast food restaurants that cater to those needs. Contrary to what you might believe, a variety of healthy foods can be found at your local convenience store, including the following:

- Low-fat milk, 100% fruit or vegetable juice, diet soft drinks, or water
- Whole-grain snacks or pretzels
- Whole-grain bagel
- Bean burrito
- Lower-fat sandwich on wheat bread
- Fresh fruit or yogurt
- Dried fruit (raisins, dried apples, or plums)
- Prepackaged salads (be careful with how much dressing you use)
- Baked potatoes or soft pretzels
- In the United States, cereal bars and graham crackers

Vending Machines

When getting a snack or drink from a vending machine, look for the following:

- 100% fruit or vegetable juices
- Low-fat milk or yogurt

*Also known as *chips* in some countries.

- Pretzels
- Cereal bars
- Raisins and other dried fruit
- Nuts

When the Food Selection Is Limited

Think of the previous week or month. How many times were you in a situation in which you didn't have control over the selection of food available to you? You might have been attending a sporting event, visiting family or friends, or taking a long road trip. Although we try to plan for these situations, sometimes they just sneak up on us. It's during these times that you may struggle to eat in a healthy manner. Try to remember that all foods fit and that learning to balance less healthy meals with other meals during your day or week is better than skipping meals. See if any of these tips will help you when you're in situations that lack a lot of food choices.

- Choose smoothies made with fresh fruit and 100% fruit juice and not fruit-flavored syrups.
- Eat only a small portion of a large cookie or cinnamon roll. You can share it with a friend or save the rest for later.
- When eating pizza, choose pizza with thin crust. If you can, order pizza with lots of vegetables and ask for half the meat and cheese.
- Buy a small bag of popcorn or peanuts instead of nachos at sporting events.

? DID YOU KNOW?

What's the "Value" in Excess Calories and Fat?

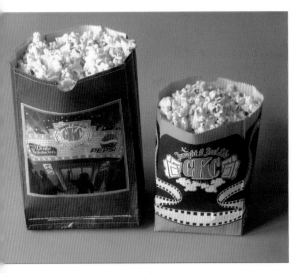

It may feel like a bargain to upgrade to a larger serving of popcorn, but it will cost you five times the calories.

Food companies are using consumers' interest in "getting a bargain" to make a profit. But our health is at risk as a result. Here's how it works. Most of the cost of food items served in convenience stores and fast food outlets is for labor, packaging, marketing, and transportation—*not* the food ingredients. So when they charge you a little more to supersize your food item, it costs them much less than the extra amount you pay. But it costs you a *lot* in terms of excess calories and fat. For example, a small popcorn upgraded to a medium costs you 23% more but adds 125% more calories! And the movie theater only spent a tiny fraction extra for the extra popcorn.

Another value-added tactic is called bundling. Say you go into a restaurant to buy a burger and a soft drink. The salesperson will try to entice you to add fries (or chips) by telling you that you'll get all three together for a little less than the cost of buying them separately. But it's not a value for your health: Instead of 640 calories for a burger and a soft drink, you would add 450 calories with the fries, for a total of 1,090 calories. And have you noticed that most fast food restaurants don't bundle the burger with a side salad, yogurt, or milk? That's because soft drinks and fries are much cheaper.

Research shows that another problem with the supersizing and bundling strategies is that the more food that is put in front of people, the more they will eat. Based on our waistlines, we don't need it!

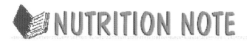

NUTRITION NOTE

May I Take Your Order?

Here's your chance to practice your eating-out skills. This activity will help you take a closer look at the differences in choices available at a quick-service food outlet. On the next page is a menu from Hal's Hamburger Heaven. Identify healthy options on the menu based on the descriptions provided. In addition, try to think of ways to eliminate high-fat condiments or ingredients to make a dish a better choice. Place a mark next to the menu items that you consider healthy choices. Write notes by any menu selections you think could be modified to be healthy choices. Answers appear on page 80.

How did you do? Go to HEED Online for a fun game that helps you identify healthy choices at many different restaurants and food outlets. See appendix C for more eating-out suggestions specific to the five HEED goals.

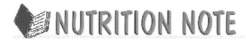

NUTRITION NOTE

Strategies for Eating on the Run

To wrap up this session, list the strategies that you have used in the past to help you make better choices at restaurants. Also add new strategies that you learned from this session that you think might help you eat better when eating out. List as many ideas as possible.

1. _____ ☐

2. _____ ☐

3. _____ ☐

4. _____ ☐

5. _____ ☐

6. _____ ☐

7. _____ ☐

Now choose two of these strategies to work on during the coming week. Place a mark in the boxes next to the two strategies you will try. Copy and post this list where you'll see it often.

Hal's Hamburger Heaven

*All prices are in U.S. dollars.

Burgers and Sandwiches

Fries, chips, or onion rings included

Cajun (Spicy) Chicken Sandwich — $4.95
Grilled or fried Cajun-spiced chicken, lettuce, tomato, onions, special sauce

Quarter-Pound Burger — $2.95
Lettuce, tomato, pickles, onions, mustard, mayonnaise

Turkey Breast Sandwich — $4.75
Lettuce, tomato, pickles, onions, mustard on white or wheat bread
Cheese extra

Half-Pound Burger — $3.95
Lettuce, tomato, pickles, onions, mustard, mayonnaise
Cheese optional

Fried Chicken Sandwich — $4.50
Lettuce, tomato, pickles, onions, mayonnaise

Grilled Chicken Sandwich — $4.75
Lettuce, tomato, pickles, onions, mustard or mayonnaise

Sides

Crispy Fries $.99 $1.25 $1.75   Baked Beans $.99 $1.25 $1.75
Onion Rings $.99 $1.25 $1.75   Baked Potato $1.25 (plain) $1.75 (loaded)

Other Favorites

Chips and Salsa — $1.75

Taco Salad — $5.75
Crispy taco shell filled with lettuce, tomato,
cheddar cheese, sour cream, and guacamole
with your choice of grilled or fried chicken

Chicken Caesar Salad — $4.95
Romaine lettuce, crispy croutons, and
grilled or fried chicken covered with
creamy Caesar dressing

Mozzarella Sticks — $2.95

Large Chicken Salad — $4.95
Lettuce, tomatoes, onions, cheese,
onion, bacon bits with your choice
of grilled or fried chicken

Side Green Salad — $2.50
Smaller version of large green salad
without chicken

Salad Dressings

Ranch, Low-Calorie Ranch, Honey Mustard, Italian, Low-Calorie Italian, French, Caesar

Drinks

Coke, Sprite, Dr. Pepper, Diet Coke $.99 $1.25 $1.50
Orange Juice $1.25 $1.75
Bottled Water $1.25 $1.75
Fresh-Squeezed Lemonade $1.25 $1.75

Session Checklist

Before you move on to the next session's activities, be sure to do the following:

- ■ Complete the Defensive Dining worksheet to determine whether you are a special occasion diner or a necessity diner.

- ■ Complete the May I Take Your Order? activity.

- ■ Complete the Strategies for Eating on the Run worksheet and try two of the strategies during the next week.

- ■ Keep track of your food intake using the Daily Food Log on a daily basis.

- ■ Visit HEED Online to learn more about healthy eating-out strategies.

We hope you've found some strategies that you can put to use right away. You've learned how to choose the healthiest options on restaurant menus and how to modify menu options to make them healthier. You've also learned how to make better choices when you're eating on the run. Try to apply some of these strategies during the coming days. In session 7, you'll learn how your thought process could affect your ability to make lasting changes in your eating habits. We'll practice replacing negative thoughts with more accurate ones.

Answers for Hal's Hamburger Heaven

Following is a list of healthy choices you could make from Hal's menu. Be sure to notice the cooking methods and preparation used of these selections. Your answers may vary based on your modifications or substitutions.

Grilled chicken sandwich	Baked beans	Side green salad
Cajun grilled chicken sandwich	Plain baked potato	Orange juice
Turkey breast sandwich on whole wheat	Taco salad with modifications	Bottled water
	Large chicken salad	

What makes these the best options on the menu? For one thing, you'll notice that we've chosen grilled (barbecued) foods such as grilled chicken sandwiches or grilled chicken salads over fried foods. Grilled foods generally have less fat and fewer calories than their fried counterparts. But beware of high-fat condiments such as mayonnaise on sandwiches and burgers. Substituting mustard for mayonnaise reduces the fat and calories in these foods. Baked beans and a plain baked potato are better options than french fries* because they provide more nutrients and have less fat and fewer calories. You can make the taco salad a healthier choice by not eating the shell and reducing or removing the cheese, sour cream, and guacamole. The chicken salad with grilled chicken and a side green salad are better options than the Caesar salad because they can be ordered with the low-calorie dressing on the side. Most Caesar salads are served with an abundance of high-fat salad dressing already tossed.

*Also known as *chips* in some countries.

SEVEN

Talking to Yourself

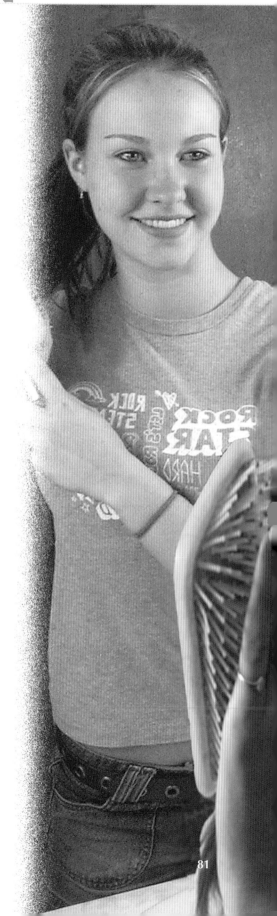

In This Session

- Understanding the interaction between your thoughts, emotions, and behaviors

- Identifying and overcoming dangerous dialogues

- Modifying your negative self-talk with positive thoughts

Pssst. We know a little secret about you. You talk to yourself. No, we won't tell the psychiatrist. In fact, talking to ourselves is something we all do. What you tell yourself can have a big impact on what you do and how you feel.

As figure 7.1 shows, your thoughts, emotions, and behaviors constantly interact. What does this have to do with healthy eating? A lot. The interaction among these components can influence your eating decisions in healthy and unhealthy ways.

Emotions drive thoughts, then thoughts drive behaviors.

1. You feel overwhelmed (emotion).
2. So you think that you don't have time to eat right (thought).
3. Then you eat haphazardly (behavior).

Thoughts drive emotions, then emotions drive behaviors.

1. You think that no one loves you (thought).
2. So you feel loneliness and self-pity (emotions).
3. Then you overeat sweets (behavior).

Behaviors drive emotions, then emotions drive thoughts.

1. You overeat at a party (behavior).
2. You feel guilty (emotion).
3. You think that you're a failure (thought).

But consider another example of this pattern:

1. You eat small portions of high-fat foods at a party (behavior).
2. You feel in control (emotion).
3. You tell yourself that you can be successful in any eating-out situation (thought).

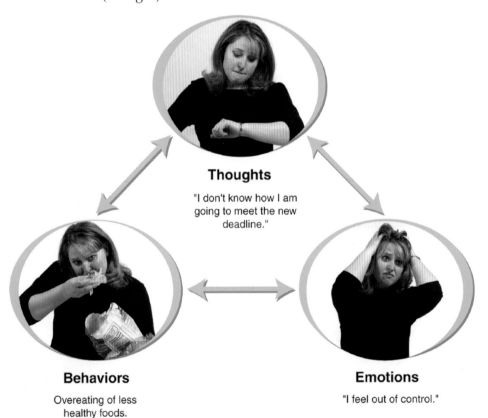

Thoughts

"I don't know how I am going to meet the new deadline."

Behaviors

Overeating of less healthy foods.

Emotions

"I feel out of control."

Figure 7.1   The thoughts-emotions-behaviors cycle. Although here the cycle starts with thoughts (thinking you might not meet a deadline), then moves to emotions (feeling out of control), and results in behaviors (binge eating), the cycle can start at any point and go in either direction.

The last example has a positive spin to it. So you see, the thoughts-emotions-behaviors cycle can be either negative or positive. It's all up to you.

Dangerous Dialogues

The "thought" part of this cycle most often starts a negative cycle. Negative thinking can lead to negative behaviors and negative emotions. Several types of negative thinking are common when people are trying to change their habits. For example, consider the following types:

All-or-none thinking is typically marked by unrealistic generalizations and often includes the words *always* or *never.*

- I can't seem to eat five servings of fruits and vegetables each day. I might as well give up.
- I always make poor choices when eating out.
- I am never going to eat ice cream again.

The problem with this kind of thinking is most apparent in the ice cream example. How realistic is it that you could give up one of your favorite foods forever? And what happens when you violate this rule the first time? Chances are it will lead to negative feelings, which may lead you to eat even more ice cream. We call this the "What the heck" effect. You definitely want to prevent this type of thinking before it starts!

Exaggerating describes thoughts that occur after a minor slip that are then blown way out of proportion to the truth. It's making a mountain out of a molehill.

- I ate the whole piece of cheesecake by myself. It must have had a billion calories.
- I haven't had any dairy foods all week. Now I'm going to get osteoporosis.

The dairy foods example is instructive. Not eating any dairy foods in a week was a slip, but one that is unlikely to affect bone health long term. Such unrealistic thoughts can discourage you and sabotage your healthy behaviors.

Faulty perceptions occur when you believe something that in reality is not true. For example, one common faulty perception is thinking that changing your eating habits is easy for everyone else but you.

- Nobody else seems to be having as much difficulty as I am. I have no willpower.
- Although I am worried about staying healthy, adopting a healthy eating pattern is just too hard for me.

Be sure to question your perceptions and make sure they are aligned with reality. Usually the truth is not nearly as bad as what we create in our imaginations!

UP CLOSE AND PERSONAL

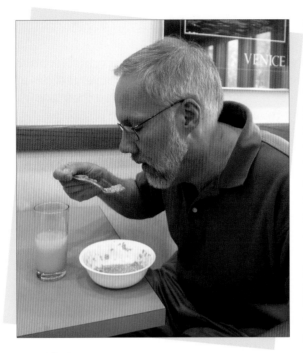

Greg joined a HEED program at his local community center because he wanted to improve his health. He thought his poor eating habits were contributing to some of his health problems. Through the assessments he did in sessions 1 and 2, Greg learned that he was eating low-fat foods most of the time and he was regularly getting two to three daily servings of dairy products. But he wasn't eating enough whole-grain foods and fruits and vegetables. Greg thought that eating most fruits and vegetables would be really hard for him. He decided that his first long-term goal would be to eat at least three servings of whole-grain foods a day.

Greg came up with two ways to achieve this goal. First, he would eat two servings of whole-grain cereal in the morning for breakfast. Second, because he took his lunch to work most days, he would switch to using whole-wheat bread for his sandwiches. Greg began to meet his goal on most days—that is, until he went on a business trip for a week. He found that restaurants rarely serve whole-grain products. Because he knew he traveled quite a bit, Greg told himself, *There is no way I am ever going to meet my goal of eating more whole grains. I might as well give up.*

Then he remembered that he had learned in HEED that such all-or-none thinking could lower his motivation to eat better. Greg quickly decided to turn his thinking around by saying to himself, *This was not a good week for meeting my healthy eating goal! I'm going to have to develop some strategies that will help me eat more whole grains while I'm on the road.* Greg took out a pen and pad of paper and started listing possible ways to get more whole grains when traveling. His list included these ideas:

- Eat oatmeal for breakfast.
- Take small boxes of whole-grain cereal with me.
- Eat low-fat popcorn as a snack.
- Take along a half loaf of whole-wheat bread to eat as a snack.
- Look for restaurants that serve whole grains, such as brown rice and whole-wheat rolls.

Greg decided that the best option for him was to choose oatmeal whenever he could. On shorter trips he would take whole-wheat bread as a snack. He figured he might not get all three of his whole-grain servings in every day, but he could come close. Greg also tried to fit more whole grain into his meals at home so that when he was traveling, he wouldn't have to be quite as vigilant. ▮

Turn Your Thoughts Around

Because the conversations you have with yourself are private, it's up to *you* to be on the lookout for negative things you say to yourself. Then you have to find ways to turn your negative thoughts into positive ones. Positive, accurate thinking will help you feel good about yourself and your efforts to eat a healthier diet.

There are three steps to stopping negative thoughts.

1. **Identify negative thoughts.** Ask yourself, *Are my thoughts having a negative influence on my feelings and actions?* Watch out for all-or-none thinking, which often includes absolute terms such as *always* and *never.*

2. **Evaluate negative thoughts.** Ask yourself whether your negative thoughts are based on truth and reality. For example, the following statement *I haven't had any dairy foods all week. Now I'm going to get osteoporosis* is not based on reality.

3. **Modify negative thoughts.** Replace negative thoughts with more positive, realistic thoughts. For example, *I haven't eaten my dairy servings this week, but I plan on restocking my refrigerator with lots of dairy options for next week.*

These steps will help you combat the negative cycle of thoughts, emotions, and behaviors. If you don't catch and correct the negative cycle, you could be headed for even more negative emotions or thoughts. You might blame yourself, have decreased self-esteem, or think that you've lost control. These all increase the chances that you'll have a lapse in your healthy eating. So it is very important that you turn the negative cycle around and get back on track as quickly as possible.

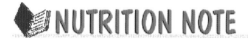 **NUTRITION NOTE**

Changing My Negative Thinking

Think of the negative statements you commonly say to yourself. Now list them on the worksheet in the blanks provided on the next page. We've provided an example for each category of negative thinking to get you started. Then use the three-step process—identify, evaluate, modify—to help turn your negative statements around.

Example: All or None Thinking

Negative thought: I can't believe I ate so much at dinner. I'm never going to be able to stop overeating!

Identify: *Never* is an absolute word.

Evaluate: I overate one time, and that does not mean I will overeat at every meal.

Modify: I'm disappointed that I overate, but I'm going to try to avoid that at my next meal. I'll dish out smaller portions and wait ten minutes before deciding whether to get a second helping. I am also going to add 15 minutes to my usual walk for the next few days.

(continued)

(continued)

Negative thought: _____

_____

1. **Identify:** _____

_____

2. **Evaluate:** _____

_____

3. **Modify:** _____

_____

_____

Example: Exaggerating or Thinking the Worst

Negative thought: "I ate the whole piece of cheesecake by myself. It must have had a billion calories!"

Identify: Does one piece of cheesecake really have a billion calories?

Evaluate: Eating one piece of cheesecake is not the end of the world and cannot undermine my entire eating plan.

Modify: I really enjoyed that piece of cheesecake. I looked it up and it only had 640 calories. I'll choose healthy food the rest of the day to ensure that I stay on track with my healthy eating plans.

Negative thought: _____

_____

1. **Identify:** _____

_____

2. **Evaluate:** _____

_____

3. **Modify:** _____

_____

_____

Example: Faulty Perception

Negative thought: "Nobody else seems to be having as much difficulty as I am in changing eating habits. I have no willpower."

Identify: "Nobody else" is a faulty statement not based in reality.

Evaluate: Other people around me have struggled with getting their eating habits on track.

Modify: Making better food choices is difficult, but the benefits will be worth it. I'll keep trying to make changes.

Negative thought: _____

_____

1. **Identify:** _____

_____

2. **Evaluate:** _____

_____

3. **Modify:** _____

_____

_____

WEIGHTY MATTERS

Does the mere mention of the words *diet* or *dieting* make you want to eat more? Researchers have found that if you normally overrestrict your food intake, just thinking about dieting can lead you to overeat. In one clinical trial, researchers studied both people who overrestrict their food intake and people who do not. When the people who normally overrestrict their eating were told they were going to be on a diet the following week, they ate significantly more during a meal than the other people in the study. This study provides evidence of the link between dieting and overeating.[14] This is one reason we promote a healthy eating pattern that you can maintain over time without "dieting."

NUTRITION NOTE

Reviewing Goals and Rewards

It has been four sessions since you set your short- and long-term goals. Now is a good time to see if you are on track toward reaching them. Take a look back at the goals and rewards you set in session 3. Have you met your goals? If so, did you reward yourself?

If you didn't meet one or more of your goals, reevaluate the goal to see if it was personal, realistic, specific, and measurable. There is nothing wrong with revising goals if they turn out to be unrealistic. Remember, Rome wasn't built in a day.

Think carefully about the goals you set in session 3 and what you have learned in recent sessions. Do you need to revise your goals? If so, use the space provided to record your new goals and rewards. Look back at your HEED pyramid assessment and HEED goal assessment in sessions 1 and 2 for ideas on areas of your diet that need improvement.

My Long-Term Goals (one month or longer)

Example: *Within six weeks, I will be eating three servings of dairy foods per day*

as confirmed by my daily food log.

(continued)

Goal 1: _____

_____

Reward: _____

Goal 2: _____

_____

Reward: _____

My Short-Term Goals (less than one month)

Example: *In the next two weeks, I will increase the number of dairy servings*

I consume by drinking a glass of nonfat milk every morning. I'll confirm this by

reviewing my daily food log.

Goal 1: _____

_____

Reward: _____

Goal 2: _____

_____

Reward: _____

Goal 3: _____

_____

Reward: _____

Goal 4: _____

_____

Reward: _____

PORTION DISTORTION

Having faulty perceptions is one way people get into negative self-talk. You can have faulty perceptions about the true size of servings, especially if you aren't familiar with measuring cups and spoons or don't have them handy when you want to know how many servings you are about to eat. Here are some easy visual reference ideas that will aid you in making sure you're eating the right sized portions. Each is for one serving.

Bread Group

1/2 cup cooked rice (80g), pasta (70 g), cereal (120 g)	Small computer mouse
Bagel	Hockey puck
Roll or muffin (1 oz or 30 g)	Plum

Fruit and Vegetable Group

Apple, orange, peach, and the like (medium whole piece)	Baseball
Dried fruit (1/4 cup or 35 g)	Golf ball
Fruit juice (3/4 cup or 180 ml)	
Leafy greens (1 cup or 55 g)	1/2 of a grapefruit

Dairy Group

Cheese (1-1/2 oz or 40 g)	6 dice

Meat Group

Meat, poultry, fish (2-3 oz, or 60-85 g, cooked)	Deck of playing cards
Nuts (2/3 cup or 90 g)	Cupped handful
Legumes (1 cup or 180 g)	Tennis ball

Session Checklist

Before you move on to the next session's activities, be sure to do the following:

- ☐ Complete the Changing My Negative Thinking worksheet.

- ☐ Review and, if necessary, revise your short- and long-term goals.

- ☐ Complete the Daily Food Log on a daily basis.

- ☐ Visit HEED Online for more information about positive thinking and healthy eating.

It is common for people who are trying to learn new habits to sometimes feel bad about how things are going. But negative thinking, emotions, and behaviors are interrelated and can affect your chances of successfully changing your eating habits. So when you talk to yourself—and we know that you do—make sure you tell yourself positive, helpful things. In the next session we turn our attention to healthy shopping strategies. We know that grocery shopping can be a daunting task for some. The tips we provide will help you master healthy shopping.

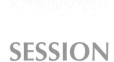

EIGHT

Healthy Shopping Strategies

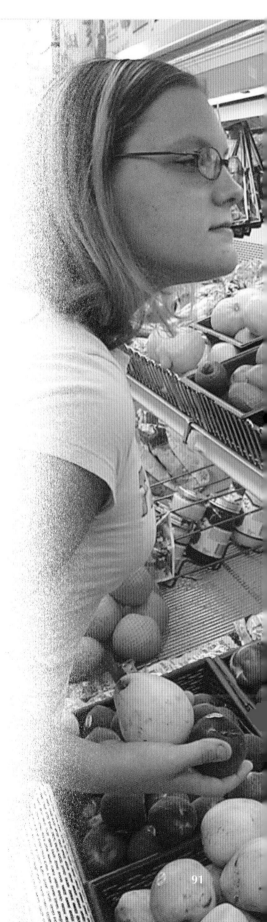

In This Session

- Overcoming obstacles to shopping for healthy foods

- Identifying the best options in each super-market department

- Using food labels to assess food choices

Nutritious meals come from nutritious ingredients. One of the first steps to eating healthier meals and snacks at home is to know how to buy healthier foods at the supermarket. Think about what foods you have in your home right now. Can you make a healthy meal out of the foods that are in your kitchen? If your answer is no, don't worry! You're not alone.

UP CLOSE AND PERSONAL

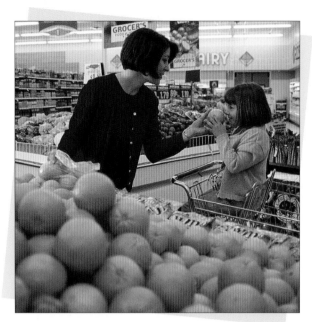

Samantha works full-time and has two very active children. When Samantha isn't working 10-hour shifts at her job, she is chauffeuring her children from soccer games to dance lessons. Samantha wants to make healthy meals for her children and herself, but she finds it difficult to keep her kitchen stocked with any food, much less nutritious food. She worries that the food her family is eating is not providing the nutrients they need.

Samantha does her weekly grocery shopping on Saturday mornings. Last Saturday was typical. She left the house without a shopping list and with only one hour to shop. She knew it was going to be a stressful trip when she couldn't find a parking spot. Then she was nearly run over by a careless shopper while she was trying to decipher the food label on a loaf of bread. She finished her grocery shopping by racing up and down the aisles, haphazardly grabbing whatever looked good, regardless of whether it was vitamin packed or fat filled.

Samantha left the supermarket feeling frustrated and disappointed. She had such good intentions! She told herself that next time she'll find a less hectic time to shop and will spend a few minutes making a list of the healthy items she needs instead of relying on her memory.

If Samantha's story and her shopping expectations sound familiar, you might need a few tips on how to better manage your trips to the supermarket. You're in the middle of making new and exciting changes to your eating habits. It's probably necessary to make changes to your shopping habits, too. Let's face it. We're more likely to eat better if we have good choices, and fewer temptations, around us. One of the best places to start is with your shopping cart! ▮

NUTRITION NOTE

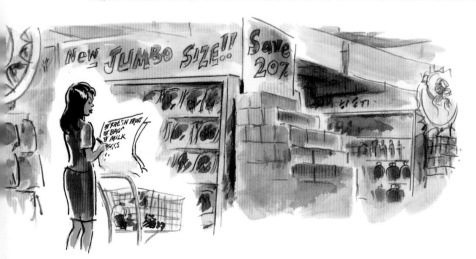

Overcoming Barriers to Healthy Shopping

Perhaps you're one of those people who will avoid the supermarket at any cost. Does it require too much time in your busy schedule? Do you hate dealing with the crowds in the store? Or maybe you feel like you're spending too much money on low-quality foods. Most of us have had one of these complaints at one time or another.

Take a look at the following common barriers to grocery shopping. We've listed some easy ways to overcome the barriers. Place a mark next to the barriers that you struggle with. Circle the solutions that you're willing to try during your next trip to the supermarket. You can also list any additional barriers you face and possible solutions in the space provided.

Barriers	Solutions
☐ Time-conscious shopper: "It takes too much time to go grocery shopping."	1. Know the layout of the store so that you can get in and out quickly. 2. Choose an unpopular time so as to avoid crowds and long lines. 3. Plan your meals and snacks in advance and make a list so that you know exactly what you need. 4. Have someone else do the shopping. 5. _____
☐ Impulsive shopper: "I never get the foods that I need to make healthy meals."	1. Make a list of the items you need, based on your recipes or meal plans. Allow yourself only one or two extra items. 2. Eat before you shop so that you're not hungry. 3. _____
☐ Kitchen-phobic shopper: "I don't like to cook, so I don't know what to buy at the grocery store."	1. Most frozen food sections contain no-prep meals and snacks. Be careful of high-fat and high-sodium foods. 2. Fruits and some vegetables require no cooking. 3. The deli often has fresh food that requires no cooking. Ask the staff if they offer healthy options or low-fat or low-calorie choices. 4. Look for a cookbook with quick and easy recipes at your local bookstore. These recipes often contain few ingredients and take less than 15 minutes to prepare! 5. _____
☐ _____	1. _____ 2. _____
☐ _____	1. _____ 2. _____

Healthy Shopping Without Breaking the Bank

You might think that you have to spend more money to eat healthy foods. This is a common misconception, but it's simply not true. In 2002 alone, Americans spent over $900 billion on food. That's an increase of nearly $40 billion from the previous year. On average, we spend about 10% of our disposable income on food each year.[15] That's not a lot, but regardless of how much you spend, you might as well get the best nutritional return for your money.

The truth is that you don't have to spend a lot of money to get a healthier payback. Remember, you are investing in your health and, therefore, in your future. Just as you may spend time and money investing in your financial future, you should also spend time investing in your health. One way to invest in your health is to budget more of your grocery money to fruits and vegetables, whole grains, low-fat foods, and low-fat dairy foods. These foods provide more nutrition value for your money! Spend less of your money on empty-calorie foods such as sweets and soft drinks, which do not give you the nutrition that you need.

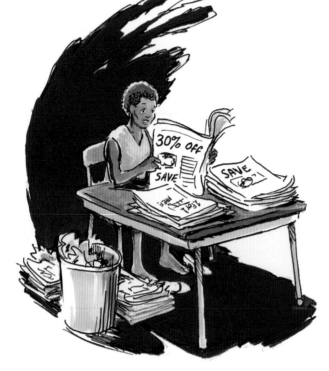

Here are a few tips to get more for your money at the supermarket:

• **Keep a shopping list and follow it when you are shopping.** When you have a list, you are less likely to impulse shop. You'll already know exactly what you need. Keep a list on the refrigerator so that your family can help you keep track of the foods that you need. Try to limit yourself to two or three impulse buys.

• **Use the newspaper inserts to find supermarket specials for the week.** Meat and poultry can be purchased when they are on sale and frozen for use at a later date. Make a special note on your grocery list of the items on sale that week.

• **Compare supermarket brands to name brand food items both for cost and nutrient value.** Many store brand foods are less expensive but have the same nutrient value as name brand food items.

• **Beware of marketing ploys such as "Buy 2 get 1 free" on items that you don't need in large supplies or that might spoil before you get a chance to eat them.** Many times these so-called sales are aimed at getting you to buy more things than you really need. The sale is a deal if you really need three of the product or if it's nonperishable. But if the food item is going to go to waste in your home, then it's really not a deal.

Maneuvering the Aisles With Ease

Maybe you can't relate to people who dislike grocery shopping. You might actually love the experience of selecting just the right produce or getting all the right ingredients for the Saturday picnic. If you're one of these people, you might just need help picking out the right types of foods in the different areas of the supermarket. Follow these easy tips for choosing the right foods from every aisle.

Breads, cereal, rice, pasta, potatoes, and corn

- When buying whole-grain breads, look for the word *whole-grain* as the first ingredient in the ingredient list. Some grain breads are not whole grains.
- Try new nonfat or low-fat baked goods. Try not to purchase products with partially hydrogenated oils as one of the first four ingredients.
- Look for whole-grain rice and pastas to use as alternatives to white rice and pasta.
- Try to buy cereals with at least 3 grams of fiber per serving. You can mix a high-fiber cereal with other cereals to enhance the taste.

Fruits and vegetables

- Buy frozen or canned fruits and vegetables when they are out of season or if you won't use them right away. Be sure to choose fruit that is canned in its own juices.
- Buy canned vegetables and rinse them with water before cooking to decrease their sodium content.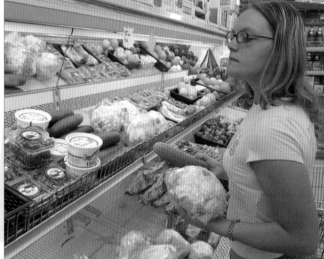
- Choose canned fruits and drain them to remove added syrups or sugars.
- Choose grapefruit and oranges that are heavy for their size. They have more juice.
- Buy fresh fruits and vegetables when they are in season because they are cheaper and higher in quality than when they are out of season.
- Buy a variety of colors of fruits and vegetables so that you get a variety of nutrients.
- If you're short of time, take advantage of convenient packaged precut salads and raw vegetables.

Dairy and dairy alternatives

- Buy nonfat and low-fat milk rather than 2% or whole milk.
- Buy nonfat or low-fat buttermilk, sour cream, cottage cheese, and yogurt in place of the regular versions.
- Buy nonfat or low-fat ice cream or frozen yogurt instead of regular ice cream.
- Watch out for yogurts with fruit on the bottom; they tend to be high in calories.
- Look for fat-free cheeses or cheeses that are made with low-fat or nonfat milk.
- Try individually packaged low-fat yogurt or yogurt smoothies, string cheese, cottage cheese, and flavored milk products when you are looking for a high-calcium snack.
- Choose low-fat, calcium-fortified soy milk products (milk, cheese, and yogurt) as healthy dairy alternatives.

Meat and meat alternatives

- Buy lean cuts of beef and pork. Look for the words *round* or *loin* for beef and *loin* or *leg* for pork.
- In the United States, choose USDA Select or Choice beef. USDA Select beef contains the least fat. Choice cuts are the second leanest.
- Buy skinless poultry or remove the skin before cooking.
- Look for frozen fish: It's less expensive than fresh fish and may be easier to find.
- Try canned (water-packed) tuna or salmon. These are great low-fat lunchtime options that can be prepared at home or away.
- Choose soy-based foods with 18 to 25 grams of protein per serving.

Snacks, desserts, and beverages

- Buy 100% fruit juices instead of fruit drinks or fruit punch.
- Choose juices high in vitamin C such as orange, grapefruit, and tomato juice.
- Look for nonfat or low-fat and low-sodium varieties of snack foods.
- Many baked desserts and crackers are made with partially hydrogenated vegetable oil. Try to limit the amount of these types of snacks.
- Warning: Just because the foods at the bakery don't have food labels that list the calorie or fat content does not mean that they are free of calories or fat!

Convenience foods

- Frozen dinners, canned foods, and prepackaged foods can be high in sodium. Their sodium content can range from 300 mg to well over 1,000 mg per serving. Aim for less than 400 mg of sodium per serving in canned foods. Try to find frozen dinners with less than 700 mg of sodium.
- Read food labels! Select low-calorie and low-fat frozen meals that provide at least 25% of the Daily Value for one or more nutrients such as vitamin A, vitamin C, iron, or calcium.
- If the frozen dinners you choose are not balanced or lack important nutrients, buy frozen vegetables or a salad that can be added to the meal.

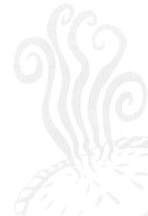 **SCIENCE UPDATE**

Each year the USDA tracks information about the amount of food available for people to eat in the United States. This food supply data can tell us a lot about trends in food purchasing and consumption. Researchers estimate that Americans ate 12% more calories per day in 2000 than in 1985. That's an additional 300 calories per day! Increased consumption of grains (mostly refined grains) accounted for 46% of the increase in calories. Added fats and sugars accounted for 24% and 23% of the increase, respectively. If you've noticed the huge number of choices in the snack food aisle of the supermarket, these data may tell us why: We're buying and eating more of these types of foods.[16]

The trends are similar in most Western nations. For information on your country's level of food consumption, see one of these Web sites:

Australia: Australian Bureau of Statistics (www.abs.gov.au)—Click on "Themes." Then find the "Health" link and then click on "Health lifestyles and risk factors."

Canada: National Institute of Nutrition (www.nin.ca)—You'll find an abundance of information relating to nutrition at this site.

Health Canada Web site (www.hc-sc.gc.ca)—This Web site provides information to help visitors make informed choices about nutrition and health.

United Kingdom: National Statistics (www.statistics.gov.uk)—Start at the "Health and care" link. Then choose the "Health" link, and then click on "Diet and nutrition and health awareness." ▌

Food Labels

Whether you love grocery shopping or not, one way for all shoppers to become smarter is to use the information that is provided on the actual food items. Food labels are found on almost every food item in the supermarket. In many countries, food labels are designed and presented in a standardized, easy-to-read format to help you make better food choices and meet your health goals. In the United States, four main types of nutrition and health information appear on the food products (figure 8.1):

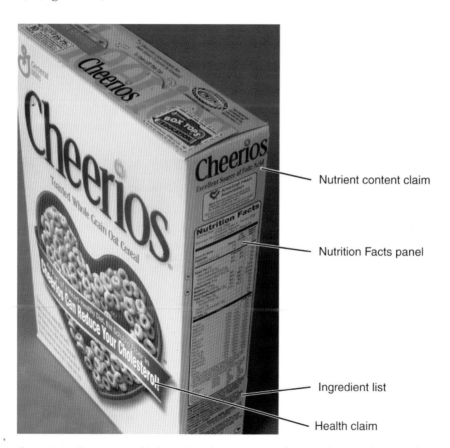

Nutrient content claim

Nutrition Facts panel

Ingredient list

Health claim

Figure 8.1   Four types of information that appear on food products in the United States.

- The **Nutrition Facts panel** provides information on calories and nutrients in one serving of a food.
- The **ingredient list** provides a list of ingredients in the food in descending order of predominance by weight. The ingredient that weighs the most is listed first, and the ingredient that weighs the least is listed last.
- A **nutrition content claim** such as "reduced fat" or "high fiber" can help you find foods that fit your nutrition needs. Foods have to meet very stringent criteria in order to put these descriptors on the food label.
- A **health claim** can be found on certain foods that are known to have potential health benefits. Health claims show a relationship between a nutrient or other substance in a food and a disease or health-related condition. Foods must meet specific qualifications to make health claims.

Getting Personal With the Nutrition Facts Panels

In the United States the Nutrition Facts panel lists nutrition information in a standard format. This panel is similar to the Nutrition Facts table in Canada, the Nutrition Information Panel in Australia, and the nutrition label or food label in the United Kingdom.

You can use the Nutrition Facts panel to help you meet your healthy eating goals. You might compare the nutrient values between two different foods, or you might read the Nutrition Facts panel to see how many calories are in one serving of a specific food. But you need to understand exactly what you're reading! There's so much information on the panel that it's easy to get overwhelmed. In figure 8.2 and the list below, we've identified the main components of the Nutrition Facts panel that can help you stay on track with your HEED goals.

- **Serving size:** The amount that makes up one serving of the food. Nutrition information applies to only *one* serving of the food.
- **Servings per container:** The number of servings in the container.
- **Calories:** The number of calories in one serving of the food.
- **Total fat:** The total grams of fat in one serving of the food. To reduce fat in your diet, look for reduced-fat or low-fat foods.
- **Saturated and trans fats:** The total grams each of saturated fat and trans fat in one serving of the food. Avoid foods that are high in these artery-clogging fats.
- **Dietary fiber:** The total grams of dietary fiber in the food. Fiber is found in whole-grain foods such as cereals, breads, and pasta. Look for foods with at least 3 grams of fiber per serving to increase your overall fiber consumption.
- **Vitamin A and vitamin C:** The percentage of your daily vitamin A and vitamin C needs. Try to choose foods and beverages with at least some vitamin A and vitamin C.
- **Calcium:** The percentage of your daily calcium needs. To increase calcium, aim for foods with at least 20% of your daily calcium needs.

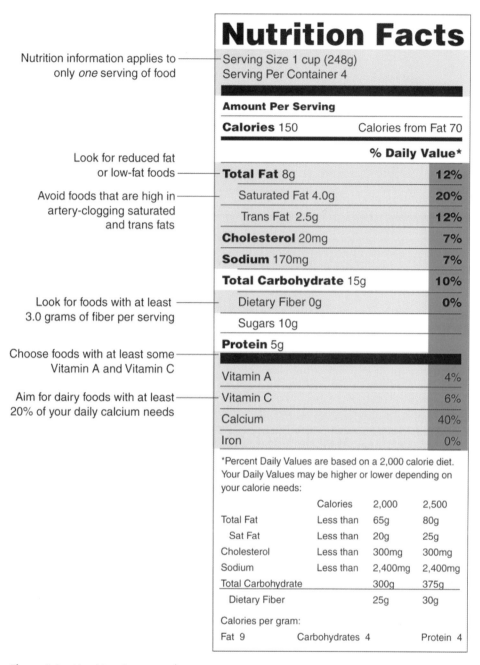

Figure 8.2 Nutrition Facts panel.

HEED Goals and the Nutrition Facts Panel

Depending on your HEED goals, you might not need or use all of the information on the Nutrition Facts panel. Table 8.1 shows you what areas of the panel we think will help you stay on track with your particular HEED goal. Notice that "Serving size" and "Servings per container" are important for everyone! Regardless of your HEED goal, you should know what a serving size is and how many servings are in the container. By knowing this, you'll be able to interpret the other information on the panel.

Table 8.1   Matching Your HEED Goals to the Nutrition Facts Panel

Nutrition Facts panel item	HEED goal				
	Increasing fruits and veg-etables	Decreasing fats	Increasing dairy and dairy alternatives	Increasing whole grains	Balancing calories
Serving size	X	X	X	X	X
Servings per container	X	X	X	X	X
Calories					X
Total fat		X			X
Saturated fat		X			
Dietary fiber	X				
Vitamin A	X				
Vitamin C	X				
Calcium			X		

Deciphering the Description

People use terms such as "light," "low," "reduced-calorie," and "fat-free" very haphazardly when referring to foods. On food labels, these nutrition descriptions actually have defined meanings. In the United States, the government regulates the use of these descriptions and verifies that they are accurate. Below you'll find a list of terms that you see on a variety of food products. Become familiar with these terms so that next time you're shopping you'll know exactly how to interpret what you're reading.

Light—The product has one-third fewer calories or 50% of the fat as that of the reference food; the sodium content of a low-calorie, low-fat food has been reduced by 50%; or a property of the food such as color ("light brown sugar").

Low—A serving contains no more than 40 calories, 140 mg sodium, 3 grams of fat, or 20 mg cholesterol.

Reduced calorie—A serving contains at least 25% fewer calories than that of the comparison food.

Free—A serving contains no or an inconsequential amount: <5 calories, <5 mg sodium, <0.5 grams fat, <0.5 grams saturated fat, <2 mg cholesterol, or <0.5 grams sugar.

High—A serving contains 20% or more of the Daily Value for a given nutrient.

High fiber—A serving contains 5 grams or more of fiber.

Healthy—A food is low in fat, saturated fat, cholesterol, and sodium and contains at least 10% of the Daily Values for vitamin A, vitamin C, iron, calcium, protein, or fiber.

Good source—The product provides between 10% and 19% of the Daily Value for a given nutrient per serving.

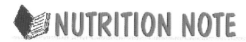 **NUTRITION NOTE**

Comparing Food Labels

Let's compare two sets of common grocery items. Although these are U.S. products, you can apply what you learn here to looking at food labels in any country. Examine the Nutrition Facts panels for the Reduced Fat Triscuit wafers and Club Crackers. Compare the serving size, servings per container, calories, total fat, saturated fat, dietary fiber, vitamin A, vitamin C, and calcium. Which of these items on the Nutrition Facts panels are different? Which product is healthier? Why?

Next, compare the Nutrition Facts panels for the nonfat and 2% milk. Circle any differences between the two. What makes nonfat milk a better option than 2% milk? Answers appear on page 104.

Reduced Fat Triscuit Crackers

Nutrition Facts

Serving Size 8 wafers (31.12g)
Serving Per Container 8

Amount Per Serving

Calories 130	Calories from Fat 25

	% Daily Value*
Total Fat 3g	**5%**
Saturated Fat 0.5g	**3%**
Cholesterol 0mg	**0%**
Sodium 170mg	**7%**
Total Carbohydrate 24g	**8%**
Dietary Fiber 4g	**17%**
Sugars 0g	
Protein 3g	
Vitamin A	0%
Vitamin C	0%
Calcium	0%
Iron	8%

Club Crackers

Nutrition Facts

Serving Size 4 crackers (14.0g)
Serving Per Container 32

Amount Per Serving

Calories 70	Calories from Fat 25

	% Daily Value*
Total Fat 3g	**5%**
Saturated Fat 1g	**5%**
Cholesterol 0mg	**0%**
Sodium 160mg	**7%**
Total Carbohydrate 9g	**3%**
Dietary Fiber 0g	**0%**
Sugars 1g	
Protein 1g	
Vitamin A	0%
Vitamin C	0%
Calcium	0%
Iron	2%

(continued)

(continued)

Nonfat Milk

Nutrition Facts

Serving Size 1 cup (240mL)
Serving Per Container 16

Amount Per Serving

Calories 90	Calories from Fat 0

	% Daily Value*
Total Fat 0g	0%
Saturated Fat 0g	0%
Cholesterol <5mg	1%
Sodium 135mg	6%
Total Carbohydrate 13g	4%
Dietary Fiber 0g	0%
Sugars 13g	
Protein 10g	
Vitamin A	10%
Vitamin C	2%
Calcium	30%
Iron	0%

2% Reduced Fat Milk

Nutrition Facts

Serving Size 1 cup (240mL)
Serving Per Container 16

Amount Per Serving

Calories 120	Calories from Fat 45

	% Daily Value*
Total Fat 5g	8%
Saturated Fat 3g	15%
Cholesterol 20mg	7%
Sodium 120mg	5%
Total Carbohydrate 11g	4%
Dietary Fiber 0g	0%
Sugars 11g	
Protein 9g	
Vitamin A	10%
Vitamin C	4%
Calcium	30%
Iron	0%

⦿ PORTION DISTORTION

As if serving sizes aren't complicated enough, you might notice that the serving sizes reported on Nutrition Facts panels don't always match the serving sizes you've learned in HEED. The HEED serving sizes are based on serving sizes defined by the U.S. Department of Agriculture. These serving sizes have been used to make national recommendations. Four factors were considered when defining the serving sizes: amounts typically reported in food consumption surveys, comparable nutrient content to other food items in the food group, easy-to-recognize household units, and serving sizes used in previous food guides. *Use the HEED serving sizes when recording your food intake to see if you're achieving your goals.*

The serving sizes that are used on the Nutrition Facts panels were established by the U.S. Food and Drug Administration. They are meant to help you compare nutrition information on similar products. They are based on serving sizes that people typically consume—*not* the recommended HEED serving size. Serving sizes on food labels should be used to compare prices, contents, and nutrient contents of various brands. They should *not* be used to track your number of servings in your daily food log.

Session Checklist

Before you move on to the next session's activities, be sure to do the following:

■ Complete the Overcoming Barriers to Healthy Shopping worksheet and try one of your solutions during your next trip to the supermarket.

■ Complete the Comparing Food Labels activity.

■ Complete the Daily Food Log on a daily basis.

■ Visit HEED Online to practice your shopping skills at the virtual supermarket.

We hope that you have learned helpful strategies to become a smart grocery shopper. Whether you do the grocery shopping for your family or not, it helps to be knowledgeable about the foods you eat. Try to put these tips into practice during the coming weeks. In session 9 we'll discuss how to enlist help from people around you. We know it's hard to make lasting changes without the support of your friends and family, and we'll show you how you can seek support.

Answers to Comparing Food Labels Nutrition Note

Differences between Reduced Fat Triscuits and Club Crackers: Serving size, servings per container, calories, saturated fat, and dietary fiber. Don't be fooled when comparing the nutrient values. One serving of Triscuits is eight wafers, while one serving of Club Crackers is only four crackers. To really compare the two, you have to double everything on the Club Crackers label! The Triscuits are a better option because they have fewer calories (for 8 crackers), less fat, and more fiber.

Differences between nonfat milk and 2% reduced fat milk: Calories, total fat, saturated fat, and vitamin C. Without question, the nonfat milk is the better option. One serving of nonfat milk has 30 fewer calories, 5 fewer fat grams, and 3 fewer saturated fat grams . . . and the same amount of calcium! It's a smart choice whether you're trying to decrease fat, balance calories, or increase dairy foods.

NINE
Recruiting Support

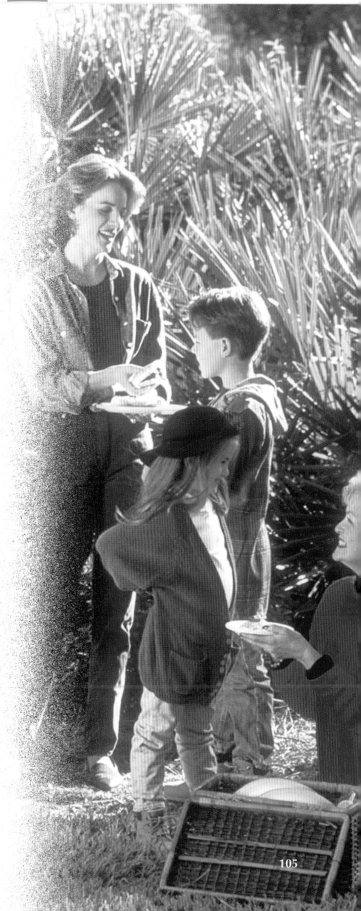

In This Session

- Identifying the types of social support you need

- Enlisting sources of support

- Recognizing people who are not supportive

You might be wondering what other people have to do with how *you* eat. Eating isn't always just about providing fuel for your body. In fact, eating often involves social or emotional aspects. For example, eating can play a central role in gatherings with friends or family. Certain foods might remind you of your childhood. And some meals mark solemn religious occasions. You are more likely to successfully change your eating habits if your family, friends, and co-workers are supportive of your efforts. If the people around you are indifferent to—or even actively oppose—your healthy eating goals, you'll have a harder time. So how do you get them on board?

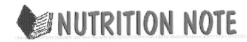 SCIENCE UPDATE

Research shows that social support is an important predictor of long-term physical activity behavior in adults. In one study, the people who had greater levels of social support were more likely to maintain their physical activity behaviors over 24 months than those who had less support. Participants who had greater levels of social support also reported having greater belief in their ability to maintain physical activity over time.[17] If the support of family and friends can help people become physically active, maybe such support can help you meet your healthy eating goals, too! ▮

NUTRITION NOTE

What Are Friends For?

Let's face it: We all need some help once in a while. Try to remember times over the past few years that you've needed support from people around you. Maybe you needed help as you were trying to change a habit, such as trying to stop smoking or increase your level of physical activity. Or perhaps you needed assistance to meet a deadline at work. In the following form, list the times when you've needed or asked for support. Identify who provided the support and how they supported you.

Times you've needed support	Who provided support and how
Moved to a new city.	New co-workers helped me find a good area to live in and introduced me to their friends.

Does this list help you see how the support of other people was important to your success? In the same way, seeking and receiving support from others will help you in your efforts to eat healthy.

Types of Support

Let's look at the different types of support you'll need as you strive to reach your HEED goals. We've given examples of each type of support. In the blanks provided, write the name of the person who might be able to give you that type of support as you work toward your HEED goals. Keep in mind that you probably won't need all types of support at once.

Listening support. People who offer listening support can listen to your triumphs and troubles without giving advice or making judgments about your thoughts or behavior. In other words, they are good "sounding boards." Listening support is helpful when you need to vent your frustrations, rehearse situations, or practice conversations. *Examples:* Advisor, friend, family member, co-worker. *My example:* _____

Shared experience support. People who have been "in the same boat" as you can be excellent sources of support. These people can relate to what you are going through. They will be able to validate many of the things you are feeling, thinking, or doing as you work to adopt a healthier eating lifestyle. They can even offer suggestions. With shared experience support, you'll know that you are not the only one facing barriers to healthy eating. *Examples:* Friend, family member, fellow HEED participant. *My example:* _____

Participatory support. People who are trying to make similar changes to you are great sources of support. Someone who makes healthy choices when you're eating out together or helps you cook healthy meals is giving you participatory support. Having this type of support helps you to be accountable to someone else for your actions. Such support might provide the extra push you need to stay on track. In addition, the social aspect of doing something together can make the whole experience more enjoyable. *Examples:* Fellow HEED participant, family member, friend, co-worker. *My example:* _____

Motivational support. This type of support is provided by people who can help increase your desire, determination, or confidence to eat healthier for a lifetime. You might think of them as coaches. They are often upbeat, energetic, and enthusiastic. People who provide motivational support may also be able to give you incentives or rewards. *Examples:* Friend, co-worker, spouse, doctor. *My example:* _____

Emotional support. People who provide emotional support help you deal with the feelings that result from trying to change. These are usually people who have some insights into your personality and your personal history. This helps them understand your difficulties and concerns. They are warm and caring in a nonjudgmental way. Consequently, they provide more than listening support. A co-worker may be a good listener, but a close friend or relative may be more likely to provide emotional support. *Examples:* Parent, child, friend, partner. *My example:* _____

Practical support. People who do things to make it easier for you to eat healthier are providing you with practical support. For example, perhaps your spouse cuts up some fruit or vegetables for you and puts them in a container so that you can then pack them for lunch.

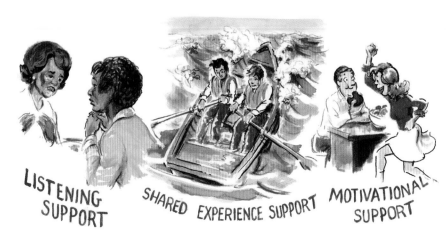

LISTENING SUPPORT   SHARED EXPERIENCE SUPPORT   MOTIVATIONAL SUPPORT

Examples: Family member, co-worker. *My example:* _____

_____

Technical support. Technical or informational support is provided by people who have expertise in the areas in which you are trying to make a change. These people can teach you about nutrition and a healthy lifestyle. They can also help you develop skills that will enable you to maintain healthy eating. Books, videos, and health professionals can be good sources of technical support. Newspapers, magazines, or television may help as well, but be careful—not all the information is accurate and unbiased. *Examples:* Books, videos, health professionals, magazines, Internet. *My example:* _____

🔍 UP CLOSE AND PERSONAL

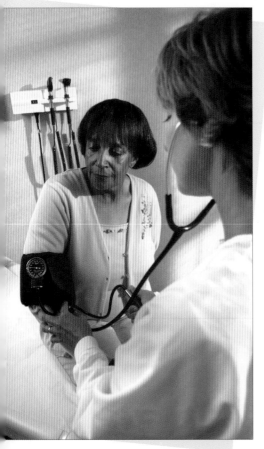

Sandra is a retired teacher who lives with her son, Ben, and her two grandchildren. During her annual physical exam, Sandra's doctor diagnosed her with high blood pressure. She told Sandra that by making meaningful changes to her eating habits and increasing her activity she could control her blood pressure without medication. When Sandra told Ben about her diagnosis, he confided that he was taking medication for high blood pressure. Together they came up with a plan for making changes to their lifestyle. They decided to cut back on eating out and to increase the number of healthy family meals that they make. Not only would this benefit their health, but it would also teach the children about making healthy choices.

Sandra was so successful in changing her eating habits that she wanted to share her success story with others. During her Monday card game, she started bringing healthier snacks and talking to her friends about the changes she was making to her lifestyle. Many of her friends had similar health problems and were really excited about making changes, too. By talking with others, Sandra had expanded her support system to include herself, her family, and her friends! She's now more confident than ever that she'll maintain her healthy changes. ▮

Building Your Support Team

It's very unlikely that one person can fulfill all of your support needs. Be especially careful about how much you ask of your spouse or significant other. Expecting that person to be all things to you can put a strain on your relationship. Think of recruiting support as building a *team* of supporters: Everyone on your team plays a role in helping you achieve your goal. For example, your spouse might be a great listener, but your best friend might be gifted at helping you in practical ways. Think about the people you interact with every day—family, friends, co-workers, and so on. Which of them would be willing and able to help you?

Enlisting support helps the people you care about be involved in the changes you're making. They might prefer this over simply *reacting* to your changes.

In addition, you'll find that as you seek support from people around you, you'll have new opportunities to support *them!* Remember Sandra's story? When she began cooking healthier meals, it improved not only her diet but also that of her family. And by providing healthier snacks for her friends, she helped to educate and motivate them to take steps toward a healthier way of eating.

Even after identifying your support team, you may still be thinking, *I can't ask my friends or family for support. I'm too strong for that.* Many people believe that asking for help is an admission of weakness. Others may fear rejection or ridicule. For whatever reason, we are not generally very skilled at asking for support. If you find it difficult to ask for support, check out the following tips. These will give you a head start the next time you need to enlist your support system.

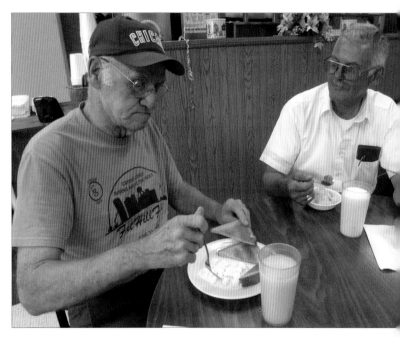

People who will eat healthy foods with you can be great sources of support.

- Define the type of support you need.
- Identify the people you can approach for help.
- Plan out your strategies for asking for help. Have back-up plans in case one of the people you approach is unable or unwilling to help you in the ways you request.
- Think of the specific ways each person can help. You need to be able to tell each person exactly what you want or need.
- Just ask! Most people will be flattered that you thought enough of them to want their help.
- Ask people how you can help them in return for their support. Together, identify ways that you can reward one another when you attain your goals.

NUTRITION NOTE

My Support Team

Recruiting people to help you change your eating habits is not easy. But learning to seek support is important if you want to make the changes easier. Remember, you probably won't have to beg for help. Most friends and family want to help! To get started, use the following worksheet to help you find ways to get the support you need to meet your healthy eating goals.

What do I need help with? What type of support do I need?	Who could help me?	How could they help?	How could I reward them for helping me?

Seeing Through Saboteurs

At times you will encounter people—even people you are close to—who are not supportive of your dietary changes. We call them *saboteurs.* Most of the time, saboteurs don't even realize that they're inhibiting your positive changes.

There are a number of reasons why someone may sabotage your healthy eating program. Your friends may feel insecure or guilty about their own eating habits, and your new changes may make these feelings worse. Your partner may feel as if your new eating habits will adversely effect how he or she likes to eat. You probably see changing your diet as a benefit, but your partner may not, especially if your partner isn't ready to make changes. Co-workers may miss the social interaction that you had during lunches at the local restaurant and feel threatened by your newfound dedication to healthy eating.

Situations like these arise quite often when you're trying to make positive changes to your eating habits. How can you cope with these dilemmas?

First, don't assume that everyone knows you're trying to improve your diet. Let the people around you know that you're working hard to change your way of eating. Try to be as honest and nonjudgmental as possible of other people's eating habits. You may tell a friend or partner that you've been thinking about making changes to how you eat for a long time and you're now ready to take steps to do it. Perhaps you've sensed cues from your body that a change is needed or your doctor has warned you about your health. Leave the door open if the other person would like to learn more about the changes you're making, but don't assume that they'll feel the same way you do. Try to reassure them that making changes to your eating habits does not mean your relationship with them will change.

Try to come up with a game plan to deal with situations that can sabotage your healthy eating plans. Whether it's a lunch out with co-workers or a party with friends, try to think of ways of dealing with these situations before they arise. This is a good time to put the IDEA problem-solving strategy to work. See pages 52 to 53 in session 4 to review the strategy.

UP CLOSE AND PERSONAL

Jesse and his wife, Mary, often travel to his Aunt Mabelle's house for Christmas. Aunt Mabelle is a wonderful cook, famous for her pies and rolls. She lives to cook for her family. It's her way of showing how much she loves them. Aunt Mabelle starts baking for special occasions weeks in advance. Jesse realizes that Aunt Mabelle would be offended if he refused to try some of her desserts, so he and Mary came up with a plan to sample one slice of her pies, but no more. If she insists that he try more than one slice, he will simply tell her, "No, thanks. I would prefer a cup of decaf coffee instead. I don't want to have too much of a great thing!" More than likely, Aunt Mabelle won't mind and all will be well. Jesse and Mary also mentally prepared themselves just in case Aunt Mabelle doesn't like their response. At least they can support each other! ▌

Session Checklist

Before you move on to the next session's activities, be sure to do the following:

- ▢ Complete the What Are Friends For? worksheet.

- ▢ Complete the My Support Team worksheet.

- ▢ Complete the Daily Food Log on a daily basis.

- ▢ Visit HEED Online to learn more about social support.

Although eating is a very personal habit, you're not in this alone! Changing behaviors is never an easy thing to do, but your support troops can help. Hopefully, you're now ready to seek help from people and move forward in achieving your goals. You're almost halfway through *Healthy Eating Every Day*. In session 10, you'll reevaluate your dietary habits to see what changes you've made. You'll have the opportunity to reassess your goals to make sure you're heading in the right direction.

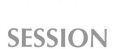

Looking Back, Looking Forward

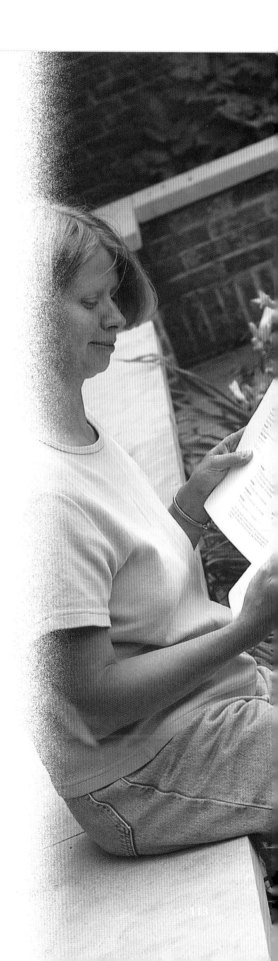

In This Session

- Learning more about the benefits of whole foods
- Evaluating your progress to date
- Setting new goals

You're halfway through *Healthy Eating Every Day!* When taking a lengthy journey, it's often helpful to pause a moment, look back to see how far you've come, and consider whether you need to adjust your course. In this session, you'll do just that. You will review the HEED goals and principles, reassess your eating habits, and set goals for the remainder of the program.

Our goal is to help you improve your health by improving the quality of your diet. The main dietary targets for HEED are decreasing fats; increasing fruits and vegetables, dairy products, and whole grains; and balancing calories. In addition, we hope you've been encouraged to eat a balanced diet using whole foods as your main nutrient sources. Whole foods are unrefined grains, beans, nuts, seeds, fruits, and vegetables. They're called "whole" because they have not been subjected to a lot of processing. In this session, you'll learn more about the importance of whole foods and their synergistic effects. You'll also have the opportunity to reassess your eating habits and revisit your short- and long-term goals.

Food Synergy

Often when it comes to foods, 1 + 1 = 3. Exciting new research is showing that two or more healthy food components often work together to achieve a health benefit that the individual components cannot achieve by themselves (figure 10.1). Let's look at one example of this.

Researchers grow cancer cells in petri dishes. Then they add certain substances to the cancer cells to test whether the substances promote or inhibit the growth of cancer cells. If the cells grow faster than normal, the substance is a cancer promoter. If the cells don't grow at all or grow more slowly, the substance is a cancer inhibitor.

In one study, scientists put cancer cells in four dishes. They didn't put anything else in dish 1. To dish 2 they added a phytochemical found in broccoli. In dish 3 they added a different broccoli phytochemical. In dish 4 they put *both* of the broccoli phytochemicals. The results? The cancer cells in dishes 2 and 3 didn't grow as fast as the cancer cells in dish 1. But the cancer cells in dish 4 grew even slower than those in dishes 2 and 3! The two broccoli phytochemicals worked synergistically to slow cancer cell growth more than the two phytochemicals did on their own. So you can see, 1 + 1 = 3.

This tells us that within certain plant foods, such as broccoli, phytochemicals work together to produce health benefits. But does synergy occur between foods from different food groups? Probably so. In the DASH study, one group of people ate a "traditional" Western diet. A second group ate the traditional diet plus 8 to 10 servings of fruits and vegetables a day. A third group ate the 8 to 10 servings of fruits and vegetables, but they also ate 3 servings of nonfat dairy foods, smaller portions of meat, more whole grains, and nuts. Compared to the first group, the second group had reduced blood pressure and blood cholesterol levels. But the third group's levels were even lower. It is likely that the added milk, and possibly the whole grains and nuts, worked

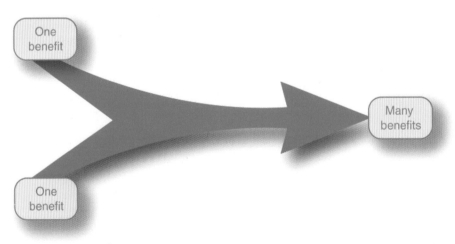

Figure 10.1   Food synergy.

together—that is, synergistically—to achieve this effect.

Food synergy is a new and exciting discovery, but scientists still have much to learn. For now, your best bet for getting the most food synergy benefits is to get your nutrients from whole foods—that is, from foods that have undergone very little processing, refining, or addition of sugar, salt, or fats. That's why four of the five HEED goal areas focus on making the best *food* choices possible.

HEED Goals Assessment: Take Two

Remember the HEED goals assessment you completed in session 2? Here's your chance to complete it again to evaluate your current eating habits. This assessment will help you see how the quality of your diet has changed over the last 10 sessions.

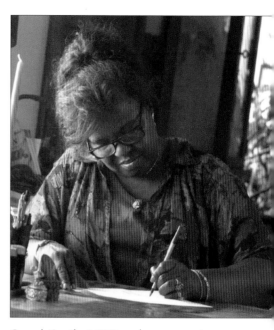

Completing the HEED goals assessment again will allow you to evaluate your current eating habits.

To take the HEED goals assessment now, go to appendix D on page 234. Photocopy appendix D and complete the HEED goals assessment by selecting one answer for each question. Read each answer carefully before choosing one. Write the score for each answer in the last column on the right. Then total the score for all questions at the bottom of each section.

As you work through each section, be sure to reflect on the following information.

• Fruits and vegetables are nutrition powerhouses. Deep orange and dark green fruits and vegetables—such as cantaloupe or rockmelon, mango, apricots, carrots, sweet potatoes, spinach, and broccoli—are excellent sources of *carotenoids*. Your body transforms carotenoids into vitamin A, which your skin, eyes, organs, and cells need in order to stay healthy. Citrus fruits (e.g., oranges, grapefruits), berries, bell peppers, papaya, broccoli, and tomato juice are all packed with vitamin C. Vitamin C helps your immune system stay healthy. It also helps your body form tissues and absorb iron from plant foods. Finally, fruits and vegetables are good sources of potassium, which helps maintain a normal blood pressure.

Bottom Line: You should choose five or more servings of fruits and vegetables per day. Are you achieving this goal on a regular basis? If not, check out the ideas in appendix C for increasing fruits and vegetables.

• Fats have the most calories of all food components. If you eat too much fat, you'll gain a lot of weight and increase your risk of certain types of cancers. Fat intake, especially of animal fats, is associated with breast, colon, and prostate cancers. Although all fats, whether from plants or animals, contain a lot of calories, the type of fats you eat can significantly influence your health. Look back at table 1.1, Tale of Two Fat Categories, on page 9. It shows the differences between the healthier unsaturated fats and the less healthy saturated and trans fats.

Bottom Line: You should choose low-fat foods most of the time. Are you achieving this on a regular basis? If not, check out the ideas in appendix C for decreasing fat in your diet.

• How did you score in the Increasing Dairy Products and Dairy Alternatives area? Research shows that dairy-rich diets may help reduce blood pressure. Interestingly, calcium alone doesn't seem to have the same effect. It appears that there is something else in dairy foods that works alone or along with calcium to reduce blood pressure. Also, despite previous recommendations, it now appears that dairy foods help *prevent* kidney stones. Nonfat and low-fat milk have the same amount of calcium and phosphorous as full-fat milk does. You won't lose much if you make the change to low-fat milk—just the heart-clogging fat and a bunch of calories.

Bottom Line: You should choose two to three low-fat or nonfat dairy servings per day. Are you achieving this on a regular basis? If not, see appendix C for ideas on increasing milk and calcium-rich foods.

? DID YOU KNOW?

Even though sour cream, cream cheese, cream, and butter are technically "dairy foods," they have little calcium and are high in fat. So they don't count toward your daily dairy group total.

Another Reason to Do Dairy

Calcium and dairy foods may have an anti-obesity effect. Studies have shown that children and adults who increase their intake of dairy foods and calcium are less likely than others to become overweight. Other studies have shown that over time, people who consume more calcium or dairy foods gain less weight than those with low intakes do. More research is needed to determine the exact way in which dairy foods affect weight, but these cutting-edge findings are exciting! Clearly, eating dairy foods is a healthy dietary strategy.

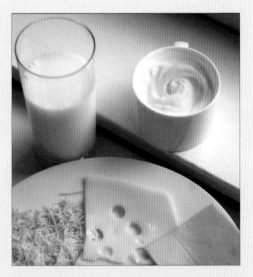

Eating a diet rich in diary products may help you reduce your blood pressure.

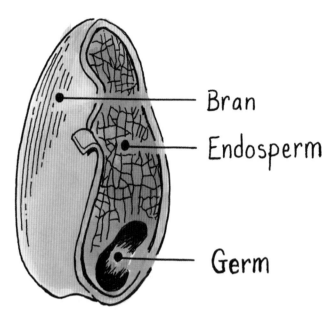

Figure 10.2 Components of a grain kernel. Refined grains do not include the bran and the germ.

• Whole-grain foods are foods whose primary ingredient is a whole grain, such as wheat, corn, oats, barley, or rice. The difference between whole-grain products and refined-grain products (such as white flour) is the manner in which they are processed. Whole-grain foods include all three parts of the grain: bran, starch, and germ (figure 10.2). But refined grains discard the bran, which is a rich source of fiber, and the germ, which contains B vitamins. Remember what we said earlier about different parts of plants working synergistically to promote health? That is likely true of the bran, starch, and germ of whole grains.

Bottom Line: You should choose at least three servings of whole-grain foods per day. Are you achieving this on a regular basis? If not, see appendix C for ideas about how to increase your intake of whole grains.

? DID YOU KNOW?

Eating more whole-grain foods may reduce your risk of colon cancer, heart disease, stroke, and diabetes. In addition, one recent study showed that women who ate more whole grains each day weighed less than women who ate few whole grains daily.[18] Scientists are trying to understand why whole grains are so beneficial. But you can't go wrong by enjoying whole grains every day.

• It's simple physics—if the calories you eat balance with the calories you burn, your weight remains stable. But if you eat more calories than you need, your body will store the excess calories as body fat. This will show up on the bathroom scale as extra weight. If you eat fewer calories than your body needs, your body fat stores will supply the needed calories, you'll have less body fat, and you'll lose weight.

If caloric balance is so simple, why are there more than one billion overweight adults globally? In modern society, it's simply too easy to eat a lot of calories and too hard to burn calories. We'll discuss increasing physical activity and controlling weight in more detail in sessions 14 and 15.

Bottom Line: You should balance the calories you eat with the calories you burn. Are you achieving this on a regular basis? If not, check out the calorie-balancing ideas in appendix C.

Now write your scores in the HEED Assessment Log in appendix A. How do your scores compare with your scores from session 2? In what goal areas did you have higher scores? Higher scores mean you have improved in those areas. Congratulations! Are there any goal areas for which you had a lower score? Don't be discouraged. You may wish to focus on these goal areas in the second half of HEED.

Balanced Diet

As you have learned, different foods have different nutrient strengths. Whole grains are high in vitamins and fiber. Fruits and vegetables are high in fiber and vitamins A and C. Most dairy foods are high in calcium and protein. And meat group foods are high in protein and the minerals iron and selenium. Although foods that are high in fat and sugar provide few nutrients, they can be a part of a healthy diet if eaten in moderation. Remember, all foods can fit.

You need to eat a balanced diet to get all the nutrients your body needs to maintain itself, prevent disease, and benefit from the synergy of foods. The Healthy Eating Every Day pyramid can be your guide to healthy eating. The whole foods, balanced eating approach is being supported by more and more research.

⚗ SCIENCE UPDATE

In one study of women, scientists identified 23 foods that were considered nutritious and consistent with current dietary guidelines (e.g., fruits, vegetables, whole grains, low-fat dairy, lean meats, and the like). They then grouped the women by the number of these foods they ate each week. The top 25% of the women ate an average of 16 of the foods. The bottom 25% ate only a little more than 6 of the foods weekly. Compared to the women in the lowest 25%, the women eating more of the healthy foods had a 31% less chance of dying early. Even women who ate a weekly average of only 10 of the foods had a lower death rate than those who ate 6 of the foods. So it doesn't take much to get a benefit.[19]

Does that mean you should panic if you had only one serving of milk today? No. When we talk about balancing your diet, we encourage you to balance it over the course of a couple of days or a week. That is, if you are low in a particular food group one day, try to eat more of the group over the next couple of days. ∎

HEED Pyramid Assessment

Now let's test whether you're getting enough of the nutrients you need. Complete table 10.1, My Daily Servings. You can use a day that you have recorded on your Daily Food Log or you can estimate the servings from a typical day.

1. For one day, beginning with breakfast, write down everything you eat and drink. Include breakfast, lunch, dinner, and snacks. If your eating patterns are not that different from day to day, you can simply think back over yesterday's food intake and write it in the space provided.

2. For each food you listed, identify the amount you ate or typically eat. Measure the amounts, if possible.

3. For each food you listed, identify the food group it belongs to (e.g., fruits and vegetables) and translate the quantity you ate into pyramid *servings*. (Use the Food Group Serving Sizes on page 11.) For each food you listed, write the number of pyramid servings you ate in the column under the food group it belongs to. For instance, if you drank 6 ounces (180 ml) of orange juice at breakfast, you would write "1" under the fruits and vegetables column, because that represents one serving size of fruit.

4. Pay special attention to how to treat the two fat groups and the sweets group. There are no standard serving sizes for these groups.
   - Place a 1 in the unsaturated fats and oils column for each time you eat any of the foods listed in table 1.1, Tale of Two Fat Categories, on page 9.
   - Put a 1 in the saturated and trans fats category each time you eat butter, stick (hard) margarine, whole milk dairy products, fatty meats, fried foods, and the like.
   - As with the fats categories, put a 1 in the sweets column every time you eat any amount of sweetened drinks, sweets, sugar, honey, cake, cookies,* pie, and sweetened desserts.

5. Finally, total the numbers in each group to view your daily intake.

To find out how your diet compares to what is recommended for you, complete tables 10.2 and 10.3. First, transfer your daily intake totals to the first column in table 10.2, labeled "My daily servings." Next, transfer your recommended servings from table 1.2, Recommended Servings for Different People, on page 12 in session 1. Then subtract what is recommended for you from your actual intake. See the first row in table 10.2 for an example. This will show you whether you are eating an appropriate amount of each food group:

- If you scored zero, you are eating an appropriate amount of that food group.
- If you scored a positive number, you are eating too much of that food group.
- If you scored a negative number, you are not eating enough of that food group.

Because there are no recommended servings for either of the fats categories, we have to treat them differently. Write your total intake of unsaturated and saturated fat in table 10.3. Then subtract the saturated and trans fat category from

---

*Same as *biscuits* in some countries.

Table 10.1 My Daily Servings

Meal	Food eaten	Amount eaten	Bread, cereal, rice, pasta, potatoes, and corn	Fruits and vegetables	Dairy and dairy alternatives	Meat and meat alternatives	Unsaturated fats and oils occurrences	Saturated and trans fats occurrences	Sweets occurrences
Breakfast									
Lunch									

Servings eaten

Dinner												
Snacks												
Servings totals												

Table 10.2   How Does My Diet Stack Up?

Food group	My daily servings	Recommended for me	Pyramid needs
Example: Fruit and vegetable group	3	5	-2
Bread group			
Fruit and vegetable group			
Dairy group			
Meat group			

From *Healthy Eating Every Day,* by Ruth Ann Carpenter and Carrie E. Finley, 2005, Champaign, IL: Human Kinetics. Organizations and agencies may not photocopy any material for professional or organizational use or distribution.

Table 10.3   Oils, Fats, and Sweets Intake

My intake		My intake	
Unsaturated oils		Sweets	
Saturated and trans fats	–		
Difference			

From *Healthy Eating Every Day,* by Ruth Ann Carpenter and Carrie E. Finley, 2005, Champaign, IL: Human Kinetics. Organizations and agencies may not photocopy any material for professional or organizational use or distribution.

Assessment 2: Session 10

HEED Goals Assessment

Date   March 12

HEED goal area	HEED goals assessment score	Change from assessment 1 to assessment 2
Increasing fruits and vegetables	21	+9 Hooray!
Decreasing fats	29	+7
Increasing dairy products and dairy alternatives	10	No change
Increasing whole grains	15	+2
Balancing calories	20	+5
Total score	95	+23 Great!

HEED Pyramid Assessment

Date   March 12

HEED pyramid group	HEED pyramid assessment score	Change from assessment 1 to assessment 2
Bread group	+1	Down from +2
Fruit and vegetable group	+1	Up from -2
Dairy group	-1	-1
Meat group	0	Down from +1
Fats	+2	Up from -2
Sweets	+1	Down from +3 Yippee!!

Figure 10.3   Example of assessment log for session 10.

the unsaturated oils. Your goal should be to end up with a positive number. In other words, you want to be eating more foods with "good" fats than foods that contain "bad" fats.

For the sweets group, enter your total intake from the sweets column of table 10.1 in the sweets row of table 10.3. Because these foods provide few nutrients and many calories, you want to keep this number as low as possible. Aim for no more than two sweets per day, especially if you're trying to manage your weight.

Record your results from the HEED pyramid assessment in the HEED Assessment Log in appendix A. Compare your current pyramid needs scores with your scores from session 1. See figure 10.3 for an example of a completed assessment log for session 10.

We will address the fats categories score soon. For all other groups, in which groups was your score a zero? This means that you are getting the right number of servings for that food group. Did you go from a negative number in session 1 to zero in session 10 in any area? If so, special congratulations to you! This means that you went from not getting enough of a specific food group to getting an adequate amount. Be careful about any food groups for which you had a number higher than zero. You may be eating more than you need for good health.

About your fats categories score: If you increased your score from session 1, you likely have made some positive changes to decrease the unhealthy fats or to increase your healthy fats. Keep up the good work. If your score went down compared to your score in session 1, try to think about ways to reduce your "bad" fats.

How about your sweets score? If you have tried to reduce the amount of sweetened drinks, sweets, desserts, and the like, you should have a lower number for your sweets score than you had in session 1. What if the number hasn't changed or has gone up? Check your food logs for ways you can substitute healthier alternatives or eliminate some of the sweets altogether.

Reviewing Goals and Rewards

These assessments have shown you what eating habits you have improved since the beginning of HEED. You probably have several areas that could still use some work. This is a good time to reset your short- and long-term goals.

Take a look back at the goals and rewards you set in session 7. Have you met your goals? If so, did you reward yourself? If you didn't meet one or more of your goals, reevaluate the goal to see if it was personal, realistic, specific, and measurable. If one or more of the characteristics of the goal is missing, you should rework the goal to include the missing characteristic. That could be the reason that you weren't successful in meeting the goal. If the goal is not personal, perhaps you should shift your goal to another area in which you are motivated to make changes. Use the HEED goals assessment and the HEED pyramid assessment that you completed in this session to identify new areas of your diet that need improvement.

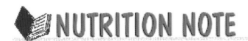

Ready? Set Goals!

The halfway point in HEED is a good time to set new goals. By taking the assessments in this session, did you learn of new areas you want to focus on? Use this form to enter new goals and rewards.

My Long-Term Goals (one month or longer)

Example: Within three months, I will increase my servings of whole grains to three servings per day as confirmed by my daily food logs.

Goal 1: _____

_____

Reward: _____

Goal 2: _____

_____

Reward: _____

My Short-Term Goals (less than one month)

Example: During the next week, I will eat one serving of whole-grain cereal for breakfast on five of the seven days. I'll confirm this by reviewing my daily food log.

Goal 1: _____

_____

Reward: _____

Goal 2: _____

_____

Reward: _____

Goal 3: _____

_____

Reward: _____

Goal 4: _____

_____

Reward: _____

Lifestyle Nutrition

The process of changing eating habits—well, any habit, for that matter—is not easy. But research has shown that using certain skills can help you change your behaviors. Setting goals is one example of an important but often-neglected lifestyle management skill. We have built many other important skills into *Healthy Eating Every Day,* some of which you have already encountered:

- **Self-monitoring your food intake.** Self-monitoring is one of the most powerful skills for changing a habit. You do this every week when you complete your food logs. As you get more experienced with monitoring, you can also keep a tally in your head of progress toward your daily goals.
- **Breaking down barriers.** Identify problem areas and then try different solutions until you come up with one that works for you.
- **Building up benefits.** As you make changes, be mindful of the benefits you are receiving. They may be as subtle as having more energy. Or they may be as dramatic as achieving a significant drop in blood pressure. Remember that some of the health benefits, such as reduced risk of heart disease, cancer, stroke, and diabetes aren't readily apparent, but they are happening behind the scenes.
- **Adjusting your thinking.** We have introduced you to the slogan "All foods can fit." Embracing this concept can help you move away from destructive "all or none" thinking. By including your favorite foods in moderation, you're less likely to binge on them.
- **Managing triggers.** Stress, boredom, happiness, yummy smells and tastes, seeing food, and certain people and events can all trigger eating when you're not physiologically hungry. You have identified your personal triggers and planned ways to deal with them.
- **Recruiting support.** Whether it's eating at home, at restaurants, or when traveling, it's easier to make lifetime nutrition changes when you have help from your friends and family. Be sure to identify people who can support you, and ask for their support.
- **Rewarding yourself.** Having more energy and better health may seem like reward enough for healthy eating. But it can take a while for some of these benefits to become evident. We have encouraged you to set small and large rewards for your short-term and long-term goals.

We'll discuss these additional strategies in coming sessions:

- **Preventing relapses.** Thinking ahead to high-risk situations for unhealthy eating and planning solutions in advance puts you in control. We'll soon show you how to recognizing brief slip-ups in healthy eating for what they are: brief departures from your goals. We'll discuss how to get back on track

  with positive action and positive thinking so that your lapse doesn't become a collapse.
- **Managing stress.** Stress is an overeating trigger for many people and can take a toll on your body over time. We will share some relaxation strategies that will help you cope with stress.

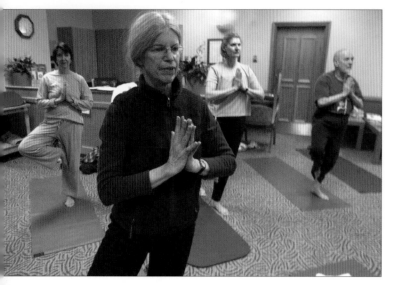

Practicing stress-reducing skills, such as yoga, can help eliminate stress as an eating trigger.

- **Managing time.** Busy schedules make healthy eating a challenge. You can control the time monster by adjusting your personal priorities. Learning quick eating options for home and away from home will also help. We'll show you how.

- **Getting confident about making dietary changes.** Nothing succeeds like success. Celebrate little achievements as well as the big ones. For example, if you used to drink three regular soft drinks per day and now you drink one, that's terrific!

Because you obtain the long-term benefits of healthy eating only if you eat in a healthy way for the rest of your life, you need to make changes that you can live with for a lifetime. All of these tools are essential for making new eating habits stick. You'll also need some nutrition-specific skills to help you along the way. In coming sessions, we'll increase your nutrition knowledge by providing tips for healthy cooking and evaluating nutrition information. We're committed to helping you eat better, so we'll continue to include these and other practical tips throughout the remainder of *Healthy Eating Every Day.*

Session Checklist

Before you move on to the next session's activities, be sure to do the following:

■ Complete the HEED goals assessment and HEED pyramid assessment and record your results in appendix A.

■ Complete the Ready? Set Goals! worksheet.

■ Go to HEED Online for a fun, interactive game that tests your skills and knowledge of HEED.

You're halfway through HEED! This is your chance to focus on learning and practicing new skills. Remember, *Healthy Eating Every Day* is just the beginning of a lifetime of healthy eating. The attitudes, skills, and strategies you learn will help you maintain your healthy eating habits for the long haul. In session 11, we'll focus on how to get back on track if you're struggling with your eating habits.

ELEVEN

Getting Back on Track

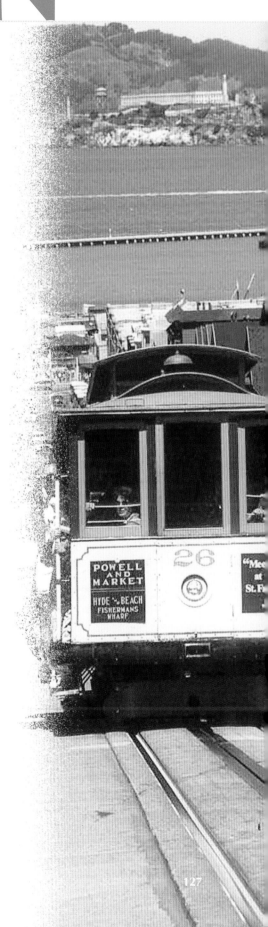

In This Session

- Preventing lapses, relapses, and collapses
- Coping with lapses when they occur

In session 10 you assessed your progress and set new goals. We hope you feel refocused and excited about the future! You have good intentions, and you've carefully developed your plans to eat healthier. Even so, you will sometimes find it difficult to make and maintain these changes. For example, you and your family may go out of town or you may take an extended business trip. At these times, making healthy food choices can be a challenge. You can be sure that disruptions in your normal healthy eating routine *will* happen.

When you're not able to stick with your healthy eating plan for a short time, we call this a *lapse.* Lapses are inevitable. But don't worry! Many strategies can prevent small lapses from completely ruining your healthy eating habits. This session will help you learn to cope with lapses so that you can maintain a lifelong healthy eating pattern.

Understanding Lapses

It's easy to think that you've blown it if you get off track in your healthy eating habits for a couple of days. This is not true! A one-time slip does not mean you're doomed to a lifetime of unhealthy eating. Missing a day or two of healthy eating is merely a short-term *lapse.* The important thing is to get back on track as quickly as possible. This will prevent a lapse from becoming a *relapse,* in which you lapse for a week or two but intend to get back on track. A relapse is more ominous than a lapse. Unless you are careful, you may easily progress to having a *collapse.* That's where you have returned to unhealthy eating habits for an extended period of time *and* you have given up the hope or desire to try to eat in a healthy manner.

Figure 11.1 illustrates the progression from lapse to relapse to collapse. It also shows some of the strategies that you can use to slow the momentum of a lapse. To eat a healthy diet for a lifetime, your first goal should be to prevent lapses from occurring. If you lapse, then you should try to prevent it from becoming a relapse. Finally, if you relapse, you should work hard to prevent a total collapse. Even if you have a collapse, don't despair: You can always return to the earlier sessions to help you get started again on your path to healthier eating habits.

Preventing Lapses

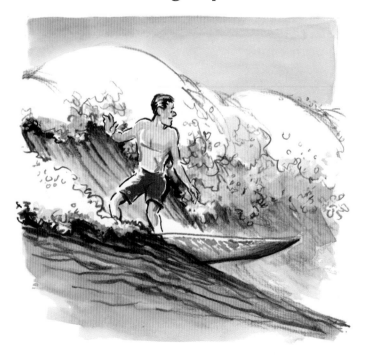

To prevent lapses, you need to nip problem eating in the bud. Following are some strategies that are especially useful for preventing lapses. These same strategies can also help you prevent relapses and collapses.

Surf the Urge

Sometimes, no matter how much you have planned in advance, an urge to eat a less healthy food choice hits you out of nowhere. An urge is like a wave in the ocean. A wave starts as a gentle swell, gets bigger and stronger as it reaches the shore, then crests and subsides. Similarly, an eating urge tends to build and build, but after a few minutes it often subsides.

Figure 11.1 Strategies to prevent lapse, relapse, and collapse.

Instead of giving in right away to the urge to eat something unhealthy, wait 5 to 10 minutes and see if the craving goes away. Try to distract yourself by moving to another room, reading a magazine, going for a walk, or calling a friend. If it doesn't go away entirely, let yourself have a small amount of the food to satisfy your taste buds.

Check Your Hunger Level

Remember what you learned in session 5: There are two types of hunger—*physiological* hunger and *psychological* hunger. When you're truly hungry (physiologically hungry), you often experience fatigue, dizziness, lightheadedness, headaches, or irritability. But psychological hunger can trick you, making you think you want to eat even though you're not truly hungry. It is usually triggered by emotions, boredom, social occasions, or the sight and smell of appealing foods. Check yourself to make sure you are eating only when you are truly physically hungry.

Plan Ahead for High-Risk Situations

Holidays, office parties, power lunches, and family gatherings are a part of our lives. You can't avoid them. Yet we know it's harder to maintain your healthier eating habits in these situations. You can still enjoy these events and minimize the risk of a lapse by planning ahead. Simply develop strategies in advance of high-risk situations so that when they occur, you are prepared to deal with them.

For example, say you plan to attend several parties around the New Year in which food will be in abundance. One way to make sure that you stay on track with your eating plan is to have a small snack before going to each party to help you avoid overeating. You can also avoid standing near the food so that you're not constantly tempted to eat more than what you had planned. Or you could add 30 minutes to your regular physical activity plan for several days to balance out the extra calories you may eat at a party. Think ahead so that you don't fall behind as you work toward your healthy eating goals.

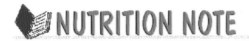
NUTRITION NOTE

Reducing High-Risk Situations

Take a few minutes to do some preventive planning. Following are four common high-risk situations for healthy eaters. As you review each situation, first think about the thoughts and feelings you might have in the situation. Then develop a plan to prevent a lapse in that situation.

Situation 1: December holidays. It's December, and your entire family is going to be visiting you. Your daily routine is likely to be interrupted. Usually in these situations, you end up eating a lot of foods that are not so healthy. You have been doing well with your healthy eating plan lately.

As someone who could potentially lapse, what are your thoughts and feelings about this situation?

_____

_____

What is your plan to prevent a lapse?

_____

_____

Situation 2: Busy at work. It's been a very busy week at work. You have an important project due, and the deadline is fast approaching. You've been working long days, but now they are going to be even longer.

As someone who could potentially lapse, what are your thoughts and feelings about this situation?

_____

_____

What is your plan to prevent a lapse?

_____

_____

Situation 3: Traveling out of town. You're going out of town for a class reunion. You will be traveling by plane and then staying in a hotel for four days. You are uncertain how you will be able to stick to your healthy eating plan during this time.

As someone who could potentially lapse, what are your thoughts and feelings about this situation?

_____

_____

What is your plan to prevent a lapse?

_____

_____

Situation 4: Outdoor holiday or vacation. It's summer, and your family is renting a cabin for two weeks. Your three children and six grandchildren are all coming. This is a fun tradition you do every summer. Your meals are usually quick and easy, and not so healthy. Snack foods are abundant. You have cake and ice cream for dessert every night!

As someone who could potentially lapse, what are your thoughts and feelings about this situation?

_____

_____

What is your plan to prevent a lapse?

_____

_____

Other situations. What other situations can you think of that may put you at risk for lapsing? A good place to start is by looking back at session 5, Tackling Triggers, to review your personal eating triggers.

_____

_____

_____

_____

As someone who could potentially lapse, what are your thoughts and feelings about these situations?

_____

_____

What is your plan to prevent a lapse?

_____

_____

_____

_____

_____

_____

? DID YOU KNOW?

Have you heard that when you crave certain foods your body is trying to tell you that you are deficient in one or more nutrients? This generally is not true. Most cravings are caused by psychological triggers such as stress, anxiety, or boredom.

Preventing Relapses

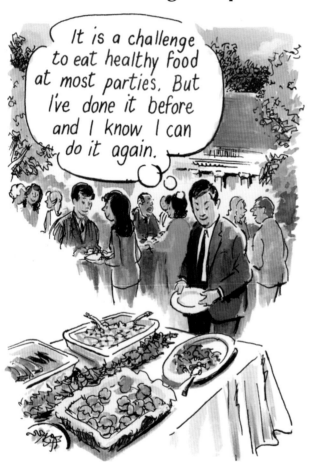

It is a challenge to eat healthy food at most parties. But I've done it before and I know I can do it again.

Despite your best efforts to prevent lapses, it is naïve to think that you will never experience a lapse. So when lapses do occur, these strategies will help you get back on track as quickly as possible so that you are less likely to relapse.

Avoid Negative Self-Talk

Avoiding negative self-talk is the most important step to take when you lapse! So often when people slip they heap negative thoughts and feelings on themselves. These bad feelings can lead to further unhealthy eating. Remember the thoughts, emotions, behavior cycle we discussed in session 7? Go back to page 83 to review the strategies for avoiding all-or-none thinking or exaggerating when lapses occur.

Monitor Your Food Intake

Have you started to get a little lazy about tracking your food intake on a daily basis? This is very common at this stage of HEED. As you have heard us say before, self-monitoring is one of the most important strategies to helping you make a change. If you find that monitoring is too hard to do all the time, it may help to simply track your food intake only at problem times—for example, at night, on weekends, when traveling, and so on. Figure out what will work best for you, make extra copies of the Daily Food Log in appendix B, and get monitoring again!

🔍 UP CLOSE AND PERSONAL

Dianne was given several new projects at work. Because of her tight schedule, she was not able to eat a healthy lunch for at least three of the past five days. By the end of the week, Dianne was feeling frustrated. Rather than give up on her healthy eating plan, she decided to start anew the following week. First, she reviewed her healthy eating benefits from session 4 to remind her why she started changing her diet in the first place. Over the weekend, she made a healthy casserole and divided it into portions to take for lunch during the week. Dianne also started monitoring her eating habits again. ▌

Preventing Collapses

If you find that you have *relapsed* in your healthy eating efforts, it is time to get serious about getting back on track. The next step could be a collapse. In addition to avoiding negative self-talk and monitoring your food intake, the following strategies will help keep you from collapsing.

Review Benefits of Healthy Eating

As time goes on, sometimes we forget why we started down a new path. You probably started *Healthy Eating Every Day* because you wanted to improve your health by improving the quality of your diet. When you relapse, review your personal benefits of healthy eating that you listed in session 4.

Reset Goals and Rewards

When you relapse, be sure to revise your goals so that they match your eating habits at the point of your relapse. For example, suppose you had gradually worked up to eating at least five servings of fruits and vegetables on all days of the week. Then you went camping for seven days, and you had a hard time fitting in your five servings. In the three weeks since your return, you have been averaging only two servings a day. Instead of going back to your pre-relapse goal of five servings seven days a week, ease up on yourself and set a smaller

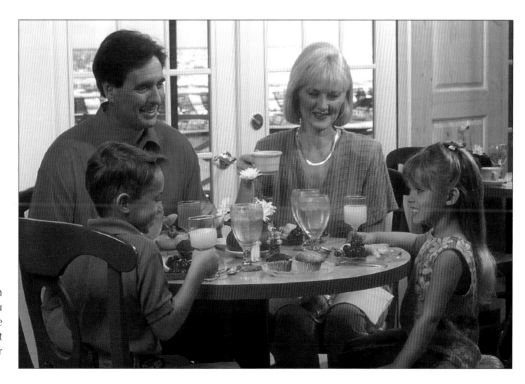

Your family can help support you when you are working to get back on track after a lapse.

goal—say, five servings at least three days a week. Then gradually set new goals to get back to your pre-relapse eating habits. Remember to use rewards to keep you motivated as you get back on track.

Renew Social Support

If there was ever a time when help from friends or family is needed, it's when you have relapsed. Remember that you can get many different kinds of support to help you get back on track. Find out who is willing to help you, in what way they can help you, and what you can do to reward them for their help. (Revisit the My Support Team worksheet on page 110 in session 9.)

⦿ PORTION DISTORTION

The French have lower heart disease death rates than Americans do. This is despite the fact that the French typically eat more fat and saturated fat than Americans eat. One possible explanation for the difference has been that the French drink more wine. Now scientists at the University of Pennsylvania and in France have found several other possible reasons for what has been dubbed the "French paradox."[20] First, researchers found that the French often package, serve, and eat smaller portions of food than Americans do. The researchers also found that although the French may eat smaller portions than Americans eat, they tend to spend more time eating—and perhaps, enjoying—their food than Americans do. So next time you think you have to eat a big meal to feel satisfied, think of the French: Take a smaller portion and eat more slowly than usual.

Session Checklist

Before you move on to the next session's activities, be sure to do the following:

- ◼ Complete the Reducing High-Risk Situations worksheet.

- ◼ Complete the Daily Food Log on a daily basis.

- ◼ Visit HEED Online to learn more about getting back on track after lapses.

Remember that lapses are going to occur. Instead of thinking of a lapse, or even a relapse, as the end of the world, think of it as a learning opportunity. Evaluate what caused you to lapse (or relapse) and use different strategies when you face the same problem in the future. Do you get much of your food from outside sources, such as restaurants, vending machines, or convenience stores? Sometimes depending on these outside sources to provide food can cause you to get off track. In the next session, you'll learn simple strategies for taking back control by cooking foods at home.

TWELVE

Cooking Up a Healthy Diet

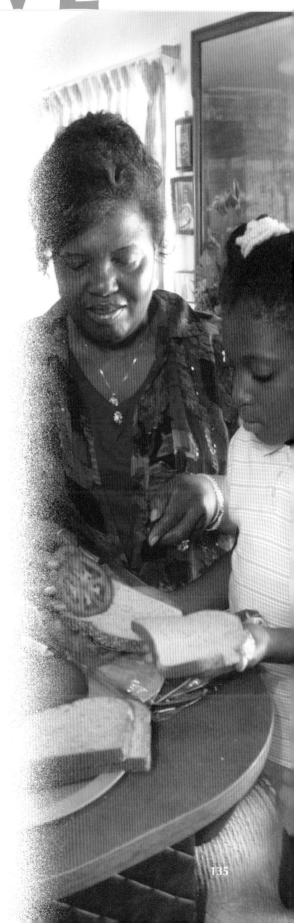

In This Session

- Understanding the role of cooking in healthy eating
- Learning how to modify recipes
- Finding ways to make healthy eating quick and easy

It's probably no surprise to you that people today are cooking much less than they did even just a generation ago. Think back over the past week: How often did you or your family prepare meals at home? If you said more than 50% of the time, you're probably in the minority among people in most Western nations. Preparing food at home has become less and less popular, sometimes because of necessity and other times because of choice.

Many factors have contributed to this change, including the following:

- **People can get cheap food quickly and easily.** As you learned in session 6, fast food restaurants, convenience stores, and vending machines offer inexpensive and convenient options when you need a fast meal or snack. Often these meals or snacks replace cooking at home.

- **Relative to the total cost of living, it is less expensive than it was 50 years ago to eat out.** Eating out at restaurants has become more affordable with the advent of eateries that accommodate families who are looking for inexpensive places to dine.

- **More women are working outside the home.** Generally in the past, it was the woman's role to prepare the meals for the family. Now that more households consist of dual-income families, fewer women have the time or the inclination to prepare meals after working all day.

- **Supermarkets offer an abundance of convenience foods.** Convenience food items such as frozen pizzas, microwavable meals, and meal-in-a-box products have a prominent place on the shelves and freezers in supermarkets. Food companies now cater to people who want to spend less time preparing foods at home.

If you still cook most, if not all, of your meals at home, you might take issue with these facts! For example, many people in the United Kingdom still cook most of their meals at home. But the influx of fast food chains and other restaurants attests to a big change in people's eating styles.

Why Cook When You Don't Have To?

If cooking isn't as popular or as necessary as it used to be, why are we spending an entire session discussing the topic? Why don't we instead think of better ways to use the space in your kitchen that is being taken up by an oven?

For one thing, cooking at home still has many benefits, such as

- better nutrition,
- more balanced meals,
- better portion control, and
- cost savings.

Cooking at home with fresh ingredients is the only way to guarantee that you have complete control over the nutritional content of your foods. The more you rely on food manufacturers for your food sources, the harder it is to achieve your healthy eating goals.

But how realistic is cooking all of your meals at home? Not very! Many people don't even know how to cook beyond microwaving. That's nothing to be embarrassed about; many people were raised in homes where cooking wasn't the norm, and others simply have no desire to know how to cook. Other barriers that often keep people from cooking at home include

- time,
- not knowing how to cook healthy foods, and
- lack of healthy recipes.

Do these sound familiar? You may even have additional barriers to cooking beyond the ones we've listed.

We're not suggesting that you have to cook all of your food from scratch in order to be healthy. Nor can we give you the skills and tools you need to be a bona fide chef. We just want to empower you to take control of your eating habits by making cooking at home a less daunting task. In this session we'll show you a simple formula for modifying recipes into healthier versions. We'll also share some tools, techniques, and tips to make healthy food preparation convenient and quick.

SCIENCE UPDATE

A recent study in the *Archives of Family Medicine* showed that eating family dinners was associated with healthy eating patterns. Compared to adolescents who didn't eat family dinners, adolescents who ate family dinners consumed more fruits and vegetables, fewer fried foods, less saturated fat, and more fiber. Now that's reason enough to stay home for dinner![21] ▮

Recipe Reconstruction

Many of us have favorite recipes that weigh in on the unhealthy side. Some are family favorites that have been passed down through the generations. Others are recipes we've collected from friends or recipe exchanges. Even though these recipes may be your favorites, they may not fit into your healthier eating pattern in their present form. Don't despair. Here are a few ways to get your recipes to "R.I.S.E." to their nutritional potential:

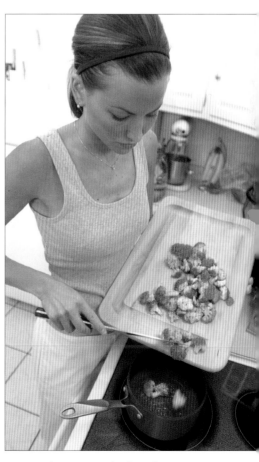

Improve the nutritional value of your recipes: Add chopped vegetables to recipes, such as adding broccoli to spaghetti sauce.

Reduce a less healthy ingredient if it is an essential part of the final product. Sometimes you can reduce ingredients in foods and barely tell the difference.

- Sugar in baked goods (reduce by one fourth to one third)
- Oil or shortening in baked goods (reduce by one fourth to one third)
- Creamy, cheesy, or buttery sauces on vegetables or in mixed dishes

Incorporate nutrient-rich ingredients. You can easily improve the nutritional value—and often the taste!—of a recipe by adding healthy foods, such as the following:

- Chopped broccoli, carrots, cauliflower, beans, or other vegetables in spaghetti sauce, tacos, sauces, soups, and salads

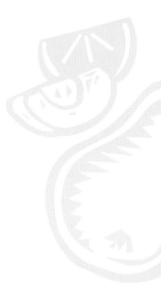

- Lots of lettuce, tomatoes, and other vegetables on sandwiches
- Powdered milk in casseroles
- Fruit in gelatin or puddings
- Tofu or soy products in stir-fry
- Wheat germ or low-fat granola (similar to muesli) in yogurt
- Whole-grain ingredients (for example, oats or whole-wheat flour) and fruits in baked goods

Substitute a healthier version of an ingredient if one is available. For example, consider the following:

- Nonfat milk in place of whole milk
- Low-fat yogurt or creamed cottage cheese instead of sour cream or mayonnaise
- Low-fat versions of cheeses and dressings
- Chicken or vegetable broth instead of gravy
- Chopped apple in place of shredded coconut in baked goods
- Applesauce instead of oil in baked goods
- Two egg whites for each whole egg (egg substitutes are another option)
- Lean ground* beef or turkey for regular hamburger
- Tofu or soy products for meat products
- Nonfat cooking spray for oil when sauteing or pan-frying foods

Eliminate a less healthy ingredient if it is optional or included primarily by habit or for appearance. For example, review the following:

- Butter or margarine on sandwiches and in mashed potatoes
- Olives in salads
- Whipped topping and frostings on desserts
- Added salt

These are just a few easy strategies for recipe repair. See table 12.1 for some other ingredient improvements.

As you modify your recipes, keep the following in mind:

- Don't change every ingredient or a large number of ingredients at one time.
- Don't expect the modified recipe to taste *exactly* like the original.
- Test the adapted recipe with various modifications until you find the version you like the best.
- Some recipes simply don't lend themselves to modification. If you find a recipe like this, or if it's a recipe that you only use on very special occasions, enjoy it in its unmodified state. Just make sure you don't use it often!

---

*Also referred to as *minced* in some countries.

Table 12.1 Ingredient Improvements

Instead of this . . .	Try this . . .	Calories saved	Fat grams saved
Dairy foods			
1 cup (240 ml) whole milk	1 cup (240 ml) nonfat milk	80	8
1 cup (240 ml) heavy cream	1 cup (240 ml) evaporated nonfat milk	621	87
1 cup (240 ml) sour cream	1 cup (240 ml) fat-free sour cream or 1 cup (240 ml) fat-free plain yogurt	347 366	48 48
4 oz. (115 g) cheddar cheese	4 oz. (115 g) reduced-fat cheddar cheese	171	25
8 oz. (225 g) cream cheese	8 oz. (225 g) light cream cheese or 8 oz. (225 g) fat-free ricotta, blended	305 621	39 87
Fats and oils			
1 tablespoon (15 ml) butter	1 tablespoon (15 ml) olive oil	*	*
1/2 cup (250 ml) oil for marinade or salad dressing	1/2 cup (120 ml) defatted chicken broth or 1/2 cup (120 ml) unsweetened pineapple juice	945 894	109 109
1 tablespoon (15 ml) mayonnaise	1 tablespoon (15 ml) reduced-calorie mayonnaise	68	11
Meat, poultry, fish, eggs			
1 lb. (450 g) ground[†] beef (80% lean)	1 lb. (450 g) 95% lean ground[†] beef or 1 lb. (450 g) ground[†] turkey breast or 1 lb. (450 g) ground[†] chicken	350 853 767	27 91 73
3 slices bacon	3 slices turkey bacon	42	5
6-1/2 oz. (185 ml) canned oil-packed tuna	6-1/2 oz. (185 ml) canned water-packed tuna	124	14
1 egg	2 egg whites	50	6

* Compared to butter, olive oil has a few more calories and fat grams, but it has 5.7 grams less saturated fat and 33 milligrams less dietary cholesterol than butter, so it is a more heart-healthy cooking choice.

†Also referred to as *minced* in some countries.

- Change is not easy. It affects not only you, but also the people close to you—your family, friends, and co-workers. Ask for their support, and show your appreciation for the support that they give you. It will help make the changes easier for all parties involved.

As you make changes to ingredients, you may need to spice up a recipe with other ingredients to add flavor. Following are some common spices and herbs used in cooking various types of food:

- *Soups:* Celery flakes, chives, black or white pepper, thyme, onion powder
- *Sauces:* Basil, bay leaves, Italian seasoning, dill weed, oregano, thyme, garlic powder, rosemary

- *Meat marinades or rubs:* Chili powder, cloves, ginger, lemon pepper, black or white pepper, sage
- *Desserts:* Allspice, cinnamon, nutmeg, cloves, pumpkin pie spice

This list only scratches the surface! The spice bottle will often list serving ideas. Don't be afraid to try new spices and keep experimenting.

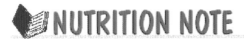

NUTRITION NOTE

My Recipe Makeover

It's time to try your hand at your own recipe reconstruction! First, pick an unhealthy recipe from your personal collection, a cookbook, or a magazine. If you don't collect recipes, think of a favorite food and ask a friend or family member for a recipe for it. Try to choose a recipe that you use often so that you'll be able to put your changes to a taste test soon. You might also keep in mind the HEED goal that you're working on.

Use the worksheet to plan the ways you could modify the recipe to make it a healthier option. Follow these steps:

1. List the ingredients and their amounts from the original recipe in the first column.

2. Record how you could modify the recipe in the next column. Refer to the list of ways to Reduce, Incorporate, Substitute, and Eliminate healthy items in your recipe.

3. Identify how the changes you propose will improve the nutritional value of the recipe. For example, your modification might reduce fat, increase fiber, increase calcium, or decrease calories.

When you've finished, give your modified recipe a try. Remember, choose one or two modifications at a time. Take notes on how your finished product turned out (too bland? too dry? just right?). You may have to try different versions of your modified recipe until you find a version you like.

My Recipe Makeover

Original ingredients	Modifications	Nutrient benefits
_____	_____	_____
_____	_____	_____
_____	_____	_____
_____	_____	_____
_____	_____	_____

UP CLOSE AND PERSONAL

Gloria loved pizza! She enjoyed the taste, and it was easy to make for her family during the week. When she started HEED, Gloria thought she would have to toss pizza from her diet. Then she discovered she could have her pizza and eat it, too! Here's how she did it:

Reduced the amount of cheese.

Incorporated many nutritious vegetables such as broccoli, spinach, tomatoes, and peppers in addition to the usual onions and mushrooms.

Substituted Canadian bacon or ham for pepperoni. Also, when she could find it at the supermarket, she used whole wheat pizza dough instead of white dough.

Eliminated the sausage and hamburger meat.

In addition, Gloria always makes sure she serves a colorful salad and low-fat milk to round out the meal. Gloria feels like she has "RISEn" to the occasion when it comes to making healthy meals for herself and her family. ▌

Finding Time to Cook

Now that you have some new strategies for preparing healthier foods at home, you need to find the time to put these strategies to work. Many of us have too little time to do the things that we enjoy on a daily basis. If you don't enjoy cooking, you might not be willing to spend even an hour preparing a meal at home. This means that you need to develop timesaving techniques that will make cooking at home possible in your busy schedule.

The following medley of timesaving tools, techniques, and tips should help you organize your kitchen for healthy eating. Put a mark beside the ones you already use. Circle two new strategies you are willing to try this week.

Tools

☐ **Slow cooker (Crock-Pot).** Makes a meal while you're away from home all day. Great for stews, tough cuts of meat, and beans.

☐ **Rice steamer.** Can cut the cooking time of rice in half. Many steamers will also keep rice warm for hours.

☐ **Storage containers.** They're great for storing leftovers and foods cooked in big batches. Purchase freezer bags and plastic containers in different sizes. Make sure they can go from freezer to microwave.

☐ **Casserole dishes.** Make a casserole on the weekend and serve it later in the week.

☐ **Blender or food processor.** They are great for yogurt and fruit smoothies, pureed bean soups, and sauces.

☐ **Grill (barbecue).** Grilling is a fast, easy, and tasty way to cook meats, poultry, fish, vegetables—even pizza! Gas grills or small indoor grills that you can keep on your countertop save the most time because you don't have to wait for the charcoal to heat up. And there are no messy pans to clean.

☐ **Freezer.** If your refrigerator or freezer is constantly crammed, think about putting a freezer in your garage or basement to hold all your make-ahead meals.

☐ **Quick cookbooks.** When choosing a cookbook with quick recipes, make sure that it also focuses on healthy recipes.

☐ **Wok.** Toss together olive oil, some lean meat, and lots of vegetables for a quick stir-fry.

Techniques

☐ Choose recipes that have five ingredients or less, with ingredients you have on hand. Don't be afraid to improvise.

☐ Cook when you have more time, for example, on weekends or days off from work. Then simply freeze, refrigerate, and reheat when time is limited.

☐ Plan weekly meals in advance. Make a shopping list and shop only once per week.

☐ Do major cooking only once or twice a week and refrigerate or freeze what you make for later use.

☐ Cook double or triple amounts. You can grill or barbecue 12 chicken breasts at once and serve some for dinner, chop up some to make chicken salad, and use the rest in soups and casseroles later in the week. Be careful: If you're not one to use leftovers, this technique can lead to a lot of waste.

☐ Gather all your ingredients and do any peeling and chopping before you start cooking.

☐ Clean as you go. You won't spend as much time cleaning after the meal.

☐ Get family members to help. They can set the table, wash vegetables, make a salad, and so on. Even young children can help out. It keeps them busy and teaches them good eating habits. As they get older, have them choose a night that they cook.

☐ For a quick pasta dish, add fresh or frozen vegetables during the last few minutes of cooking the pasta. Drain and top the pasta and vegetables with your favorite sauce.

☐ Try stir-frying. If you don't have a wok, a large, heavy frying pan will work. Use frozen vegetables, frozen shrimp, or chopped lean meat, poultry, or fish. It's an easy way to make a "one-pot" meal in minutes.

Tips

☐ Make a hearty soup or a colorful salad for your main course. Add a whole-grain roll, a glass of nonfat milk, and a bowl of frozen berries for dessert. What a balanced meal!

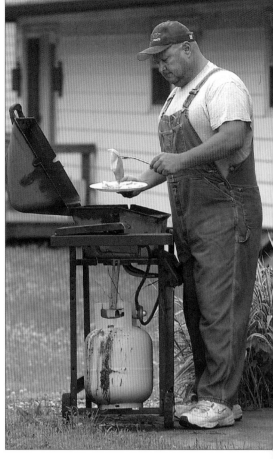

☐ Most frozen dinners, no matter how healthy they proclaim to be, lack balance. Complement the quick meal with a salad or vegetable and a glass of nonfat milk.

☐ Set out breakfast for the next morning as you clean up dinner.

☐ Prepare lunches the night before.

☐ Eat simple breakfasts, such as ready-to-eat cereal, frozen waffles, or smoothies, during the week. Save pancakes, French toast, and omelets for leisurely weekends. If you make extra waffles or muffins on the weekends, you can freeze them for use during the week.

Stocking Your Kitchen

To cook healthy meals, you have to have the right ingredients on hand. As you grocery shop over the next few weeks, consider stocking up on these dry goods and frozen items. By having these ingredients in your cupboards and freezer, you'll be better able to cook up healthy meals at home.

Grilling or barbecuing is fast and healthy.

For your cupboards
- Canned tomatoes
- Canned beans
- Whole-grain pasta, brown rice, and other whole grains (bulgur, kasha, barley, and the like)
- Low-fat sauces
- Healthy broths and soups
- Fat-free bread crumbs
- Heart-healthy oils, such as olive and canola
- Your favorite herbs and spices

For the freezer
- Frozen vegetables (be adventurous, but skip the ones with high-fat sauces)
- Fruits (look for ones that don't have sugar added)
- Skinless, boneless chicken breasts
- Fish without breading
- Low-fat filled pastas such as tortellini or ravioli

Session Checklist

Before you move on to the next session's activities, be sure to do the following:

- ■ Complete the My Recipe Makeover worksheet and try your modified recipe.

- ■ Try two new timesaving cooking strategies.

- ■ Complete the Daily Food Log on a daily basis.

- ■ Visit HEED Online to get more tips about preparing food at home.

By cooking at home, you are in control of the ingredients that go into your meals. You don't have to be a professional chef or a dietitian to turn home cooking into healthy cooking. You can use some of the simple strategies we've shown you in this session to cook up a healthy diet quickly and easily. In the next session, you'll learn how to distinguish nutrition facts from fads. You'll also learn the latest information on dietary supplements.

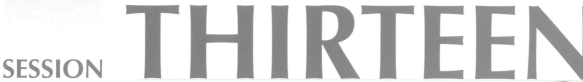

THIRTEEN

Dietary Supplements and Fad Diets

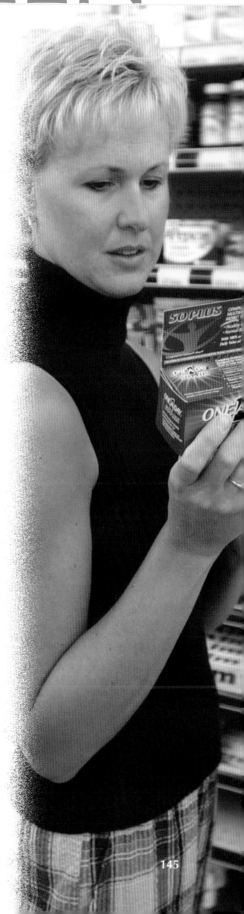

In This Session

- Deciphering the truth about dietary supplements and fad diets

- Evaluating nutrition information

Reports about dietary supplements and fad diets are news media staples. Sometimes we hear about their benefits, and sometimes we hear about their drawbacks. With so much information out there, how can you distinguish the truth from the hype? In this session, we will help you sort out the facts behind popular dietary supplements and fad diets. We'll also give you guidelines to help you evaluate nutrition information.

Dietary Supplements

Next time you're at the pharmacy or supermarket, stroll down the dietary supplement and vitamin aisle. You may be surprised by the number of bottles you see, let alone the number of them with names you can't pronounce. Welcome to the world of dietary supplements! If you're like most people, you don't know exactly what a dietary supplement is and what it's supposed to do for you. A dietary supplement is a vitamin, mineral, herb, botanical substance, or amino acid that is ingested with the intent of *supplementing* the diet. Dietary supplements are not intended to replace the nutrients that you get from food.

You're probably familiar with some common vitamin or mineral supplements, such as multivitamins or calcium supplements. In fact, you may be taking one! Herbal supplements such as echinacea, ginseng, and St. John's wort are commonly advertised because of their claims to boost immunity, decrease memory loss, or lessen anxiety. Amino acid supplements such as L-glutamine are not as well known. They are popular among people trying to improve their physical fitness. Some claim that L-glutamine increases muscle growth and stamina. Although these claims may not be supported by sound research, consumers are left with the responsibility of judging the information for themselves. We're here to help you do just that.

? DID YOU KNOW?

The following essential vitamins and minerals can be found in many of your favorite foods.

- **Vitamin C:** Oranges, kiwi, strawberries, green and red peppers, broccoli, spinach, tomatoes, potatoes
- **Vitamin E:** Wheat germ, nuts, vegetable oils
- **Beta carotene:** Carrots, sweet potatoes, winter squash, red and orange peppers, tomatoes, papayas, cantaloupe (rockmelon), apricots, watermelon, mango, spinach
- **Folic acid:** Green leafy vegetables, cabbage, nuts, eggs, whole-grain cereals
- **Vitamin B$_6$:** Meat, cereal, grains
- **Vitamin B$_{12}$:** Meat, fish, poultry, eggs, milk (animal products)
- **Calcium:** Milk, cheese, yogurt, broccoli, calcium-fortified products

Why Take Supplements?

Choosing whether to take a dietary supplement should not be taken lightly. It can be difficult to know which supplements, if any, are right for you. Certain groups of individuals should definitely consider taking supplements:

- Women who might become pregnant should take a supplement of folic acid to reduce the risk of birth defects.
- Some older adults are encouraged to take a supplement of vitamin D and calcium to reduce the risk of osteoporosis.

- People who are lactose intolerant should take a calcium supplement containing vitamin D to prevent bone loss.
- Strict vegetarians should take a vitamin B_{12} supplement to prevent anemia, which can result from the lack of meat sources in their diet.
- Individuals who are on a very low calorie diet may need a multivitamin to ensure adequate intake of vitamins and minerals.

If you eat a balanced diet, you'll likely get the nutrients you need. But research shows that multivitamins can be a healthy part of a balanced nutrition plan. You can take a standard multivitamin so that you're sure to get enough vitamins and minerals even when you're not making the best food choices.

Look for these things when choosing a multivitamin:

- Make sure the multivitamin contains vitamins and minerals close to 100% of the Daily Values (DV).
- Avoid multivitamins that contain more than 100% of added vitamin and mineral doses. You can have too much of a good thing!
- Check the expiration date. Don't buy a supplement whose date has passed.
- Multivitamins that use the word *natural* to describe their ingredients are not significantly different from standard multivitamins. Don't buy a multivitamin just because you see the word *natural* on the label.
- Make sure the label states that the multivitamin has passed the 45-minute dissolution test. This means that the pill will dissolve, and your body will absorb the nutrients, in a timely manner.

Nearly 65% of adults are not consuming the recommended amount of calcium from food sources.[22] If you fit into this category, consider taking a calcium supplement with vitamin D. These important nutrients are needed to prevent bone loss. You might also want to focus on the goal of increasing your intake of dairy products for the remainder of HEED.

What Are the Risks?

Although some dietary supplements are safe, some can have terrible side effects (table 13.1). For many supplements, it's too early to know whether they work or have side effects. In the United States, the Food and Drug Administration

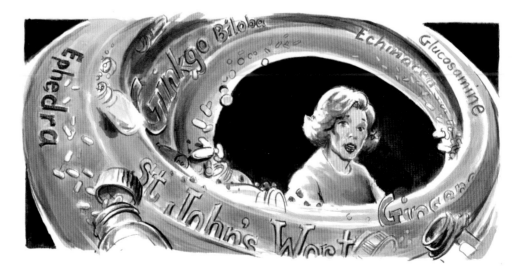

Table 13.1   Herbal Supplements Effectiveness and Safety

Herb	Claim	Effectiveness and safety concerns
Echinacea	Boosts immunity.	Unproven benefits. Do not use if you have tuberculosis, multiple sclerosis, or an autoimmune disease!
Ephedra (ma huang)	Speeds up metabolism, which promotes weight loss.	Does not effectively aid in weight loss. Increases heart rate and blood pressure and may cause stroke. Do not use if you have diabetes, hypertension, or heart disease! May cause insomnia, seizures, and possibly death. **Beginning in the spring of 2004, the FDA in the U.S. has banned all sales of ephedra and products containing ephedra because of the unreasonable risk of illness or injury.**
Ginkgo biloba	Helps prevent memory loss and reduces anxiety.	A few studies have shown some limited, short-term benefits for Alzheimer's patients. Do not use if taking a blood thinning medication. Large doses may cause nausea, vomiting, and dizziness.
Ginseng	Boosts energy; improves athletic performance.	Inconclusive and unproven benefits. Do not use if you have high blood pressure. May cause insomnia, menstrual problems, and diarrhea.
St. John's wort	Helps prevent anxiety, depression, and insomnia.	Unproven benefits. Recent research shows that St. John's wort is ineffective in treating depression. Do not take with prescription medications before checking with your doctor. Avoid use if in sunlight.
Creatine	Aids in muscle building and increases energy stores.	May help athletes train more intensely, but has not been shown to improve the duration of exercise. Adverse reactions may include nausea, muscle cramping, and some minor stomach distress.
Glucosamine and chondroitin	Help reduce pain from osteoarthritis and other types of arthritis.	No conclusive evidence. May cause nausea or indigestion. Possible blood-thinning effects.

(FDA) has advised consumers to be wary of taking supplements under certain conditions. Some supplements cause ill effects when taken with prescription and over-the-counter medicines. For example, Coumadin (warfarin, a prescription drug), Ginkgo biloba (an herbal supplement), aspirin, and vitamin E can thin your blood. Taking them together or in various combinations can increase the risk of internal or excessive bleeding.

Some supplements can have unwanted effects during surgery. These effects can be severe, especially if your doctor is unaware of your supplement use. It's crucial that you tell your doctor about your use of vitamins, minerals, herbs, or any other supplements you are taking before your surgery. Your doctor may ask you to stop taking these products at least two weeks before the procedure. Doing so will help avoid interactions such as changes in heart rate, increased bleeding, or increased blood pressure.

Table 13.1 shows only a few popular examples of the many vitamin, mineral, and herbal supplements. Remember that a supplement of any type can be harmful if not taken carefully. Only a few of them can legitimately claim to have positive effects proven by sound scientific research. Always check with your doctor before taking any type of supplement and even before taking a multivitamin. **A well-balanced diet is best!**

? DID YOU KNOW?

Reporting Adverse Events

In the United States, the FDA monitors adverse events and illnesses caused by dietary supplements. If you experience a serious adverse event, notify the FDA immediately:

Phone: 800-FDA-1088

Fax: 800-FDA-0178

Web site: www.fda.gov/medwatch/how.htm

Fad Diets

As with dietary supplements, fad diets continue to make headlines almost daily. Fad diets are weight-loss plans that often use drastic measures to help you lose weight. You may have heard of the spinach soup diet, the low-carbohydrate diet, and the blood type diet, in which you eat specific foods for your blood type. These are all fad diets. Such diets and diet books often pop up overnight and gain popularity through word of mouth.

Fad diets often produce results at first, but they don't provide lasting benefits. Because they require drastically reducing caloric intake in some way, they often do result in weight loss. But the minute you start eating more calories than your body needs (that is, you stop following the diet), you gain back the weight you've been trying so hard to lose. All fad diets are lacking in some way.

UP CLOSE AND PERSONAL

John has struggled with his weight since his early twenties. As a child and teenager, John was very active in sports and extracurricular activities. He didn't realize how many calories he was burning doing all these activities. He enjoyed eating whatever he wanted without thinking twice about his weight.

Things changed when John went away to study at a university. Instead of playing basketball and soccer, he was stuck in the library studying or working on projects for

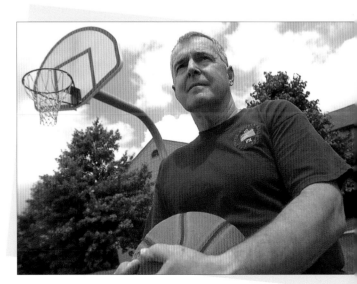

school. It didn't help that the only activity his part-time job required was working his fingers on a calculator. The weight slowly began to add up. Eventually John found himself 40 pounds (18 kg) overweight by the time he was 30.

Since then he has tried every diet imaginable, even one where he could eat only vegetable soup! He got down to his previous weight several times but was never able to maintain the weight loss for more than a few weeks.

Finally, on his 50th birthday, John decided that he'd had it. He wanted to lose the excess weight for good. He knew he needed to improve his health. He remembered that one of his co-workers had lost a large amount of weight a few years back and had managed to keep it off. He decided to ask her how she had done it.

Amy was flattered that John had asked for her advice on improving his health. She explained to John that she, too, had tried every diet imaginable and had failed completely. She had finally decided that she needed to make a commitment to her health before she'd be successful. Amy enlisted the help of a registered dietitian to help her learn how to eat a balanced, healthy diet. She also joined a walking club. John knew he didn't have the extra money to spend on a dietitian. Amy offered to share her information and tips with John to help him start eating a balanced diet. They also began eating lunch together to help keep each other on track. John has gradually lost 10 pounds (4.5 kg) and feels invigorated by his new lifestyle. He has even joined an older adults basketball league to help the weight loss process along! ∎

Deciding If a Diet Is Unhealthy

Have you experienced the yo-yo effect of fad dieting? In some cases, you may not have even realized that you were on a fad diet because it may have been disguised by unproven health claims. How do you know what is fact and what is fiction? The following characteristics can help you identify unhealthy diets. (Keep in mind that what the diet claims to do may not be what the diet actually does.)

- Promotes weight loss that is dramatic and rapid—more than 1 to 2 pounds, or 0.5 to 1.0 kg, per week
- Promotes very low calorie eating that lacks essential vitamins and minerals
- Results in fatigue (because of nutritional inadequacy)
- Does not promote lifestyle changes related to eating and physical activity
- Does not provide scientific evidence to support claims, or the "evidence" is based solely on personal testimonies
- Does not inform users of the dangers and health risks associated with the diet
- Does not provide weight maintenance ideas when the diet ends

If two or more of the statements apply, the diet is probably a fad or unhealthy diet. Remember: If it sounds too good to be true, it probably is!

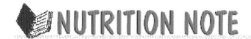
NUTRITION NOTE

Fact or Fiction?

Following are descriptions of two diets. Use the criteria provided in the previous list to evaluate the diets. List the characteristics of the diet that helped you identify them as fad diets.

Diet 1

Sarah has been on a new diet for the past month. She saw the infomercial for the quick weight-loss diet on late-night television. She was immediately hooked by the amazing before-and-after pictures, even though she wasn't sure about the credentials of the "researcher" explaining the diet. The eating program is rather boring. Sarah eats nothing but cabbage soup for lunch or dinner. But she's lost over 10 pounds (4.5 kg). She's feeling run-down, so it's good that she doesn't have to incorporate any physical activity to lose weight.

_____

_____

_____

_____

_____

_____

Diet 2

Randall has finally found something that works for him. He loves eating meat, but his meat intake had been restricted by his doctor because of its saturated fat content. On this new diet, as long as he stays away from fruits, vegetables, and grain products, he's free to eat whatever type and amount of meat he wants. No more worrying about low-fat meats and cheeses or trying to watch every small amount of margarine he uses. Randall couldn't believe his eyes when he lost 5 pounds (2.3 kg) in the first week. All those success stories on the Internet must have been true!

_____

_____

_____

_____

_____

_____

❓ DID YOU KNOW?

Low-Carbohydrate Diets

One of the most popular and longest-lasting fads has been the low-carbohydrate diets. These are diets that instruct people to eat large amounts of high-protein foods—mostly meats and poultry—and to restrict carbohydrates (grain foods, fruits, and vegetables). People lose weight at first because they are restricting their overall intake of food and because they lose a lot of water weight. Low-carbohydrate diets have many names, but some characteristics are universal to them all. These diets are unhealthy because they

- lack variety and therefore don't provide adequate nutrients (very low in fiber, vitamins, minerals, and phytochemicals);
- are high in cholesterol and saturated fat (although blood cholesterol levels may drop at first, people who use high-protein diets for a long time may be at increased risk of heart disease);
- may increase risk of developing gout, a painful disease that affects the joints;
- may impair kidney function; and
- have not been shown to promote weight loss for the long term.

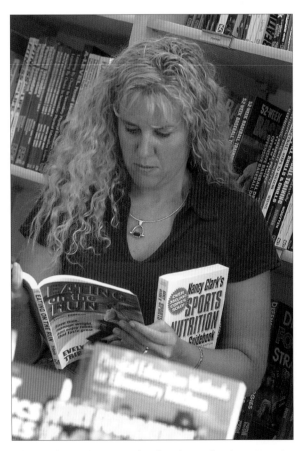

When selecting nutrition books, choose books written by reputable authors who cite scientific sources.

Identifying Nutrition Misinformation

Not all the information you hear about nutrition is true. You may turn on the TV and hear that drinking five glasses of juice a day is the most nutritious diet. Then the next day you might read a magazine article telling you that juice is too high in sugar and drinking it is a surefire way to gain weight. What do you do? Who do you believe? Whether you're seeking information about a dietary supplement, a fad diet, or nutrition advice in general, you need to know how to sort out the truth. Many different people have many different opinions. You should choose wisely whom you listen to. Here are a few ways to make sure the information you receive is valid.

- Check the credentials of the author or source. The person should have a degree in nutrition or a health-related field. The author should be associated with a reputable hospital, university, or research institute.
- The material should be relatively current because scientific information changes often based on new research findings.

- Be a skeptic. Does the information make sense compared to what you know of basic nutrition principles?
- References from valid sources should be cited. Scientific journals are the most valid of sources. References to them are often found at the end of a document. For instance, you can find the references we used in this book on page 239.

We realize that identifying nutrition misinformation can be difficult. That's why we've provided a list ("Healthy Eating Resources") of sources of sound, reliable nutrition information on the HEED CD-ROM. This list of resources can serve as a starting point for answering some of your nutrition questions. Consider these additional tips if you are trying to identify misinformation:

- Be wary if immediate, effortless, or guaranteed results are promised.
- Look for telltale words and phrases such as "breakthrough," "miracle," "secret remedy," "exclusive," and "clinical studies prove that . . ." without references to scientific journals.
- Beware of promotions for a single product claiming to be effective for a wide variety of ailments.
- Don't forget that, unlike scientists and health professionals, quacks do not subject their products (including diets) to the scrutiny of scientific research. The quack simply thrusts a product onto the market in order to get your money.
- Be cautious of money-back guarantees; a guarantee is only as good as the company that backs it.
- Again: If it sounds too good to be true, it probably is!

Session Checklist

Before you move on to the next session's activities, be sure to do the following:

- ◼ Complete the Fact or Fiction? activity.
- ◼ Complete the Daily Food Log on a daily basis.
- ◼ Visit HEED Online to get more tips about supplements and fad diets.

In this session you learned about dietary supplements, fad diets, and evaluating nutrition misinformation. We hope you're now better able to assess the nutrition information you hear or see. In all of the sessions so far, we've been looking at eating habits. In session 14, we'll shift gears and discuss the benefits of physical activity. If you're interested in balancing calories, you'll find a lot of help in sessions 14 and 15.

Answers for Fact or Fiction?

Diet 1: Rapid weight loss, very low calorie diet, fatigue, no physical activity, no scientific evidence, and sounds too good to be true.

Diet 2: Rapid weight loss, lacks essential nutrients, no warning about health risks, supported by testimonials but not scientific evidence, and sounds too good to be true.

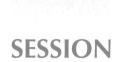

FOURTEEN

Balancing Calories With Physical Activity

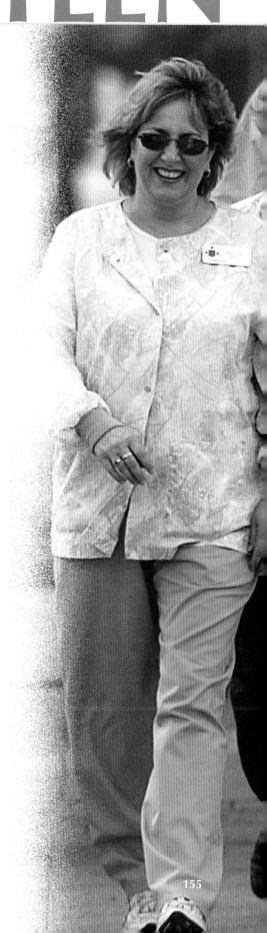

In This Session

- Understanding the benefits of regular physical activity

- Dispelling myths about physical activity

- Planning ways to become more physically active

As you will see in the next two sessions, the balance of calories between what you eat and what your body burns determines whether you gain, lose, or maintain weight. Even though it's as simple as that, overweight and obesity are rapidly growing beyond epidemic proportions in most developed countries. Balancing calories is obviously more difficult than it seems.

If you already enjoy an active life, good for you! This session will help reinforce what you're already doing. If you are a couch potato or active only every once in a while, we'll give you tips to help you start moving toward better health.

Be Fit to Benefit

One of the most important benefits of physical activity is that it can help you manage your weight. But there are plenty of other reasons to get active. Regular physical activity provides tremendous health benefits. Recent studies at The Cooper Institute have shown that if you are unfit, you are as likely to die an early death from cardiovascular disease as are people who smoke.[23] In addition, compared to people who are unfit, being moderately or highly fit can add six to nine years to your life.[24] And if you are physically active and fit, you're less likely than others to face disability in your later years.[25]

The following lists show some of the many benefits of exercise. Put a mark beside the ones that matter most to you.

Improves

☐ bone strength

☐ immune function

☐ mood

☐ self-esteem

☐ muscle strength

☐ heart and lung function

☐ flexibility of muscles and joints

☐ balance and coordination

☐ ability to do daily activities

Decreases

☐ blood cholesterol

☐ blood pressure

☐ risk of heart disease

☐ risk of diabetes

☐ risk of obesity

☐ risk of certain cancers

☐ stress

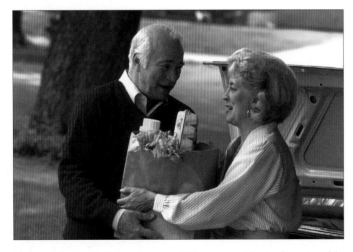

By staying physically active, you'll be more able to do enjoyable activities well into your older years.

Clearly, being physically active and getting fit is powerful medicine for both mind and body. It's not simply nice to do if you can fit it in. Rather, it's something you need to make a regular part of your lifestyle.

I Can't Exercise Because . . .

If exercising is so good for you, why don't more people do it? We're very familiar with the reasons why people aren't physically active. Can you relate to any of these?

- **I don't have time.** This is the number one reason cited for not exercising. We are frazzled by too many job, family, and community activities. The good news is that you don't have to exercise for hours to benefit. At least thirty minutes a day is what's recommended. Even better news is that you don't have to do it all at once. You can walk for 10 minutes during your break at work, ride bikes with your kids for 10 minutes after dinner, and spend 10 minutes digging a new flower bed.

- **I can't afford a gym membership or equipment.** You don't have to join a health club or have fancy home gym equipment to get active. Shopping malls, bike paths, parks and nature preserves, dance halls, gardens, and flower beds are just some of the many free or inexpensive exercise "equipment" options available to you. Of course, if you want to join a health club, that's great too!

- **I'm too old (or frail) to exercise vigorously.** It's never too late to start living an active life. Studies have shown that previously sedentary 80-year-olds improved their ability to get up from a chair and walk without a walker after starting an exercise program. Being active can help maintain your body's strength and prevent disease as you age. You don't have to exercise vigorously to get health and fitness benefits. You can do moderate-intensity activities such as brisk walking, dancing, and energetic vacuuming. Or try golfing without a cart, washing and waxing your car by hand, and raking leaves. Anything that feels similar to a brisk walk (as if you're rushing to get somewhere because you're late) will count. If you have a chronic medical condition or are concerned about increasing your activity level, contact your doctor for guidance.

- **I was an athlete in high school.** Unfortunately, fitness does not last unless you continue to be active. The health benefits of physical activity cannot be stored. You have to be active on a regular basis for your entire life to reap the benefits.

- **I don't like to exercise.** This is an easy one. Simply do what you like to do and build physical activity into it. Do you like to watch TV? Get up during the commercials and walk around, or ride an exercise bike while you watch. Do you like to shop? Walk a few laps around the mall before you start shopping. Do you enjoy spending time with friends after work? Meet at a park and walk instead of sitting on a barstool.

- **I don't know how to get started.** Read on!

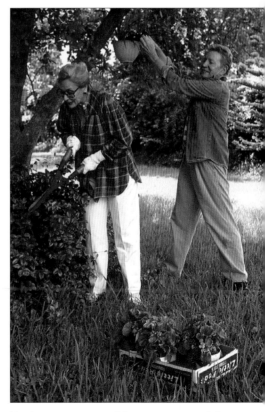

You're never too old to get up and be active!

? DID YOU KNOW?

The U.S. Surgeon General recommends that all Americans accumulate at least 30 minutes of moderate-intensity physical activity on most (preferably all) days of the week. You don't need to live in the United States for this advice to apply to you! If you currently meet these standards you may get additional benefits—especially weight management benefits—by becoming more physically active or including more vigorous activity. In other words, *some* physical activity is better than none, and *more* is even better.

🔬 SCIENCE UPDATE

Getting Steps the Old-Fashioned Way

Scientists at the University of Tennessee asked 92 men and women of an Old Order Amish community to wear step counters for a week.[26] Step counters, or pedometers, are small devices that count the steps one takes while walking. As in most Amish communities, the primary occupation of the study group was farming, which is done with horses rather than tractors. They do not use electricity, gas-powered vehicles, or other modern conveniences. The average number of daily steps in this study was 18,425 for men and 14,196 for women. That is two to three times what most people who use modern technologies get! Of the study participants, 26% were overweight. This is less than half the rate of the U.S. population today. This creative study supports the notion that we lead much more sedentary lives than that of our ancestors 150 years ago. This inactivity has probably contributed to the growing obesity problem. ∎

Finding Opportunities

There's no doubt about it: Getting active takes effort. Our modern world conspires against us by all the labor-saving devices that we take for granted. To get more active and burn more calories you have to find ways to move more and sit

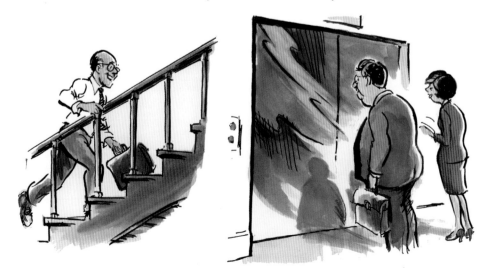

Choosing physically active alternatives is an effective way to add physical activity to your day.

Table 14.1 Which Labor-Saving Devices Can You Replace With a Physically Active Alternative?

Labor-saving device	Physically active alternative
Riding in subways, busses, cars	Walking
Using elevators and escalators	Taking the stairs
E-mailing or phoning a co-worker	Walking to a co-worker's office
Using self-propelled and riding lawn mowers	Cutting the grass with a hand mower
Gathering leaves with a leaf blower or vacuum	Raking leaves
Using a drive-through car wash	Washing and waxing the car by hand
Using a remote control	Raising the garage door by hand
Using a remote control	Getting up and turning the TV channel by hand
Driving a cart when golfing	Walking the golf course
Using a power saw	Cutting a board by hand

less. That's often easier said than done. One way to start is to choose more active options when labor-saving options are available. Table 14.1 shows a few of the many ways you could fit more activity into your everyday routines.

SCIENCE UPDATE

The Cooper Institute recruited sedentary men and women and randomly assigned them to one of two groups: the *structured exercise* group and the *lifestyle exercise* group.[27] The structured exercise group received a six-month membership to our state-of-the-art fitness center. They also had access to staff to help them plan their exercise programs. After the six months were over, participants were asked to exercise on their own for another 18 months.

The people assigned to the lifestyle exercise group met for 60 minutes once a week for six months. In those meetings, they learned lifestyle management skills that could help them begin and maintain a physically active life. For example, they learned about setting goals and rewards, self-monitoring, seeking support, and thinking positively. The lifestyle exercise group did not exercise during the meetings but learned how to build moderate-intensity activities into their lifestyles as best they could. After six months, the group met less regularly over the final 18 months of the study.

At the end of 24 months, both groups had significantly increased their physical activity and fitness levels and improved numerous health parameters. The average results of the two groups did not differ from each other. This means that the lifestyle exercise approach is an effective alternative to a more traditional, structured exercise program. Joining a gym is very good, but it's not the only way to get active! The study also found that people who increased their use of the lifestyle skills were more likely to be maintaining their higher level of activity several years after the study than were those who did not use the lifestyle skills. Researchers have also found that the lifestyle approach seems to be more cost-effective than the structured exercise approach.[28] ∎

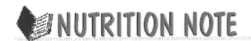 **NUTRITION NOTE**

Strategies for Getting Active

Whether you want to increase your activity to get healthier, to lose weight, or both, you can take many paths to live an active life. We'll outline three strategies here to help get you started.

Strategy 1: Reduce the amount of time you spend in sedentary activities. Sedentary activities are activities in which you're sitting or lying still. For example, you could go for a walk after dinner instead of settling in for a night of TV. In the space provided, list three sedentary activities you do frequently. Estimate how much time each day you spend doing each one. After you complete the list, select one sedentary activity that you will try to spend less time doing in the next week. Circle the activity and write in how you are going to decrease it. For example, you might replace it with a more active pursuit.

Sedentary activity	Minutes per day	How I will do less of this
_____	_____	_____
_____	_____	_____
_____	_____	_____

Strategy 2: Increase the intensity of your light activities by doing them more vigorously. For example, instead of strolling at the mall, you might make it a brisk walk. Your body will benefit, and you'll get your shopping done a lot faster! Other examples might include mowing the lawn or washing the dishes. In the space provided, list three light-intensity activities you do often. Estimate how much time each day you spend doing each one. Select one that you will increase to moderate intensity in the next week. Circle the activity and write in how you are going to increase it.

Light activity	Minutes per day	How I will increase the intensity
_____	_____	_____
_____	_____	_____
_____	_____	_____

Strategy 3: Add moderate-intensity activities to your day. Ten 2-minute brisk walks add up to 20 minutes of exercise! In the space provided, list the times when you could add a 2- to 5-minute walk into your day. Try to think of everything—the commercials during television shows, time during your coffee breaks, or a longer route to the bathroom or lunch. Circle at least one that you will try this week.

Walk opportunities

1. _____   4. _____

2. _____   5. _____

3. _____   6. _____

Next Steps

Are you inactive but interested in learning more about how you can become more active and fit? If so, check out the *Active Living Every Day* program. This program is based on The Cooper Institute study described in this session. It is made available through Human Kinetics at www.ActiveLiving.info or by calling 800-747-4457. You can also order step counters by calling this number. Many people find that step counters motivate them to move more.

UP CLOSE AND PERSONAL

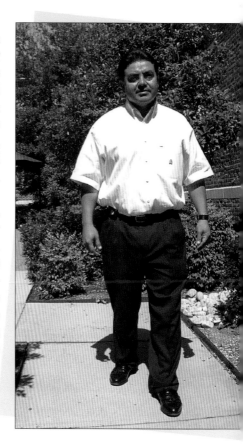

Carlos received a step counter for his birthday from his friend Jill. Jill had been wearing a step counter for several months. She found that it really motivated her to be more physically active. Jill told Carlos that he should wear it all day long and aim for at least 10,000 steps a day. Carlos wisely decided to see what his usual step count was before he jumped right in to going for 10,000. He wore it for seven days without changing his usual activity level. Was he in for a surprise! He averaged only 3,745 steps per day.

Initially disappointed because he had so far to go, Carlos set a short-term goal to increase his activity level by 500 daily steps each week. At first it was hard because he wasn't used to thinking about being more active. But whenever Carlos noticed the step counter on his belt, it would remind him to look at it. He would then plan his activities for the day around his step count. If his step count was low, he created ways to get in more steps. He walked to co-workers' offices instead of e-mailing them. He walked to local restaurants for lunch, and he took his dog on longer walks after getting home from work. Each night he recorded his total steps on the computer.

Gradually, he increased his steps to just over 10,000 a day. He was pleased to have reached the goal. He was even happier when his blood pressure went down and his doctor reduced the dosage of his medicine. Carlos found that the simple step counter helped him set goals, monitor his physical activity, and feel motivated to be more active. ∎

Session Checklist

Before you move on to the next session's activities, be sure to do the following:

- ▪ Complete the physical activity benefits checklist at the beginning of this session.

- ▪ Complete the Strategies for Getting Active worksheet.

- ▪ Complete the Daily Food Log on a daily basis.

- ▪ Visit HEED Online to learn more about increasing your physical activity level.

We have only scratched the surface when it comes to helping you improve your physical activity habits. Still, you should have enough information to begin to plan ways to become more active. You can apply some of the skills you have learned in HEED to help you become a lifelong exerciser. Goal setting, rewards, social support, positive thinking, planning for high-risk situations, and daily monitoring are useful strategies no matter what habit you're trying to change. In session 15, we'll help you understand more about successfully controlling your weight. You'll learn how energy balance affects weight management. And you'll get a chance to reassess your HEED goals.

FIFTEEN

Controlling Weight

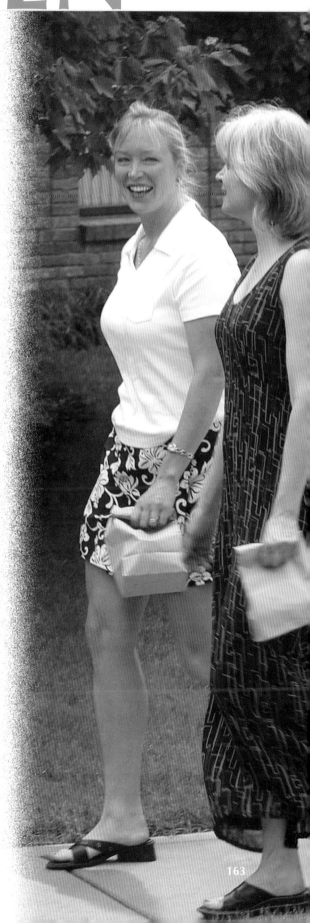

In This Session

- Understanding your body mass index and what it means for your health

- Learning about energy balance and weight management

- Reassessing your HEED goals

By now you've probably changed some of your eating habits. That's great! You may have started thinking about making changes in other areas, too. Changing your eating habits will not automatically lead to changes in other parts of your life. That's why in session 14 you learned about the role that physical activity plays in a healthy lifestyle. We hope you'll be able to start incorporating physical activity into your daily life. This session will build upon that topic to explore the area of weight control.

If you read the paper or watch the evening news, you know that weight management is a hot topic. It goes beyond fad diets and miracle cures. In fact, it's very serious. Reports from U.S. national surveys indicate that 65% of Americans are overweight and 31% are obese.[29] In Australia, about 37% are overweight and only 15% are obese.[30] While in England, about 40% of adults are overweight and about 22% are obese. This has big implications for all of us. Studies have shown that health care costs for individuals who are obese are vastly higher than the costs for normal weight individuals. In fact, health care costs for people who are obese are even higher than health care costs for smokers.[31] These statistics confirm the need for more sound information on weight control. Nearly 40% of Americans are on a diet or trying to lose weight, but often they experience poor long-term results.

Can you relate? Have you tried to lose weight but experienced the frustration of gaining it back again? You are not alone. In this session, we'll

- help you better understand the terms *overweight* and *obese,*
- explore the idea of *energy balance*—the key to weight management,
- identify the factors that affect weight gain, and
- identify characteristics of successful weight-loss programs.

By the end of the session, you'll be armed with knowledge and practical tips for how to take control of your weight and improve your overall health. You'll also reassess your HEED goals in preparation for the last five sessions.

Body Mass Index

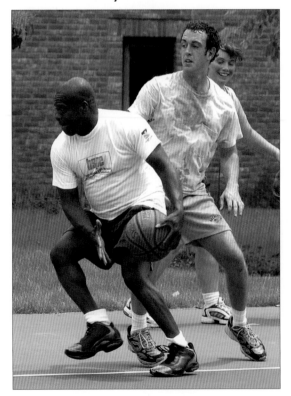

If you're slightly overweight but still physically fit, you have a lower risk of death than do people who are normal weight but unfit.

Perhaps you've heard the term *body mass index (BMI)*. BMI is, quite simply, the ratio of a person's weight to height. It's a way of quickly assessing the risk of obesity. Scientists and health professionals around the world use a person's BMI to determine if the person's weight is considered healthy for his or her height.

The World Health Organization has classified BMI values into four main weight categories:[32]

- BMI less than 18.5: *underweight*
- BMI between 18.5 and 24.9: *normal weight*
- BMI between 25 and 29.9: *overweight*
- BMI of 30 or greater: *obese*

Why are these categories important to keep in mind? Research has shown that a BMI of 25 or greater is associated with increased risk for chronic diseases such as heart disease, diabetes, and even some types of cancer. When it comes to BMI, knowing which category you fit into may help you better understand your overall health status.

NUTRITION NOTE

Finding My Body Mass Index

It's easy to calculate your BMI. Use the BMI chart on page 166 (figure 15.1). Find your height across the top and your weight on the left side of the chart. If you use the metric system, find your height across the bottom and your weight on the right side of the chart. The point where your height and weight intersect on the chart is an estimate of your BMI.

Fill in the blanks with your current weight, BMI, and BMI category.

My weight: _____ My BMI: _____ My BMI category:_____

Now think back to your weight 5 and 10 years ago. Look at the chart to see what your BMI was during those years. Fill in the blanks with the appropriate weight, BMI, and BMI category.

10 years ago

My weight:_____ My BMI:_____ My BMI category:_____

5 years ago

My weight:_____ My BMI:_____ My BMI category:_____

Are you surprised by your results? Has your weight changed over the last 10 years? Has this weight changed which BMI category you fit into? If your answer is yes to any of these questions, statistics show that you're in the majority rather than the minority. This session will help you identify ways that you can take control of your weight and your health.

You can calculate your BMI in a more detailed way in session 15 of HEED Online at www.ActiveLiving.info.

? DID YOU KNOW?

It's helpful to know your BMI because it's a popular measure to classify weight. But you should also consider other factors when assessing your weight. BMI assesses only your weight-to-height ratio; it doesn't completely account for your body composition. Perhaps you fit into the overweight category according to your BMI, but you're an avid weightlifter and physically fit. You may be an athlete with well-developed muscles, or you may have a larger, denser body frame than some people. Either of these situations could cause you to weigh more compared to others that are your same height. On the other hand, you may fit into the normal BMI category but have an excess of body fat because you have poor eating habits or you're not physically active. This could mean that you're still at risk for some diseases. You could lower your risk by eating a healthier diet and increasing your physical activity. Remember that disease prevention is about improving overall health, not just losing weight!

Figure 15.1 Body Mass Index

Height in inches

Wt. (lb)	48	49	50	51	52	53	54	55	56	57	58	59	60	61	62	63	64	65	66	67	68	69	70	71	72	73	74	75	76	77	78	Wt. (kg)
100	30.6	29.3	28.2	27.1	26.1	25.1	24.2	23.3	22.5	21.7	20.9	20.2	19.6	18.9	18.3	17.8	17.2	16.7	16.2	15.7	15.2	14.8	14.4	14.0	13.6	13.2	12.9	12.5	12.2	11.9	11.6	45.5
105	32.1	30.8	29.6	28.4	27.4	26.3	25.4	24.5	23.6	22.8	22.0	21.3	20.5	19.9	19.2	18.6	18.1	17.5	17.0	16.5	16.0	15.5	15.1	14.7	14.3	13.9	13.5	13.2	12.8	12.5	12.2	47.7
110	33.6	32.3	31.0	29.8	28.7	27.6	26.6	25.6	24.7	23.9	23.0	22.3	21.5	20.8	20.2	19.5	18.9	18.3	17.8	17.3	16.8	16.3	15.8	15.4	14.9	14.5	14.2	13.8	13.4	13.1	12.7	50.0
115	35.2	33.7	32.4	31.2	30.0	28.8	27.8	26.8	25.8	24.9	24.1	23.3	22.5	21.8	21.1	20.4	19.8	19.2	18.6	18.0	17.5	17.0	16.5	16.1	15.6	15.2	14.8	14.4	14.0	13.7	13.3	52.3
120	36.7	35.2	33.8	32.5	31.3	30.1	29.0	27.9	27.0	26.0	25.1	24.3	23.5	22.7	22.0	21.3	20.6	20.0	19.4	18.8	18.3	17.8	17.3	16.8	16.3	15.9	15.4	15.0	14.6	14.3	13.9	54.5
125	38.2	36.7	35.2	33.9	32.6	31.4	30.2	29.1	28.1	27.1	26.2	25.3	24.5	23.7	22.9	22.2	21.5	20.8	20.2	19.6	19.0	18.5	18.0	17.5	17.0	16.5	16.1	15.7	15.2	14.9	14.5	56.8
130	39.8	38.1	36.6	35.2	33.9	32.6	31.4	30.3	29.2	28.2	27.2	26.3	25.4	24.6	23.8	23.1	22.4	21.7	21.0	20.4	19.8	19.2	18.7	18.2	17.7	17.2	16.7	16.3	15.9	15.4	15.1	59.1
135	41.3	39.6	38.0	36.6	35.2	33.9	32.6	31.4	30.3	29.3	28.3	27.3	26.4	25.6	24.7	24.0	23.2	22.5	21.8	21.2	20.6	20.0	19.4	18.9	18.3	17.8	17.4	16.9	16.5	16.0	15.6	61.4
140	42.8	41.1	39.5	37.9	36.5	35.1	33.8	32.6	31.5	30.4	29.3	28.3	27.4	26.5	25.7	24.9	24.1	23.3	22.6	22.0	21.3	20.7	20.1	19.6	19.0	18.5	18.0	17.5	17.1	16.6	16.2	63.6
145	44.3	42.5	40.9	39.3	37.8	36.4	35.0	33.8	32.6	31.5	30.4	29.3	28.4	27.5	26.6	25.7	24.9	24.2	23.5	22.8	22.0	21.5	20.8	20.3	19.7	19.2	18.7	18.2	17.7	17.2	16.8	65.9
150	45.9	44.0	42.3	40.6	39.1	37.6	36.2	34.9	33.7	32.5	31.4	30.4	29.4	28.4	27.5	26.6	25.8	25.0	24.3	23.5	22.9	22.2	21.6	21.0	20.4	19.8	19.3	18.8	18.3	17.8	17.4	68.2
155	47.4	45.5	43.7	42.0	40.4	38.9	37.5	36.1	34.8	33.6	32.5	31.4	30.3	29.3	28.4	27.5	26.7	25.8	25.1	24.3	23.6	22.9	22.3	21.7	21.1	20.5	19.9	19.4	18.9	18.4	17.9	70.5
160	48.9	47.0	45.1	43.3	41.7	40.1	38.7	37.3	35.9	34.7	33.5	32.4	31.3	30.3	29.3	28.4	27.5	26.7	25.9	25.1	24.4	23.7	23.0	22.4	21.7	21.2	20.6	20.0	19.5	19.0	18.5	72.7
165	50.5	48.4	46.5	44.7	43.0	41.4	39.9	38.4	37.1	35.8	34.6	33.4	32.3	31.2	30.2	29.3	28.4	27.5	26.7	25.9	25.1	24.4	23.7	23.1	22.4	21.8	21.2	20.7	20.1	19.6	19.1	75.0
170	52.0	49.9	47.9	46.6	44.3	42.6	41.1	39.6	38.2	36.9	35.6	34.4	33.3	32.2	31.2	30.2	29.2	28.3	27.5	26.7	25.9	25.2	24.5	23.8	23.1	22.5	21.9	21.3	20.7	20.2	19.7	77.3
175	53.5	51.4	49.3	47.4	45.6	43.9	42.3	40.8	39.3	38.0	36.7	35.4	34.2	33.1	32.0	31.0	30.1	29.2	28.3	27.5	26.6	25.9	25.2	24.5	23.8	23.1	22.5	21.9	21.3	20.8	20.3	79.5
180	55.0	52.8	50.7	48.8	46.9	45.1	43.5	41.9	40.4	39.0	37.7	36.4	35.2	34.1	33.0	32.0	31.0	30.0	29.1	28.3	27.4	26.6	25.9	25.2	24.5	23.8	23.2	22.5	22.0	21.4	20.8	81.8
185	56.6	54.3	52.1	50.1	48.2	46.4	44.7	43.1	41.6	40.1	38.7	37.4	36.2	35.0	33.9	32.8	31.8	30.8	29.9	29.0	28.2	27.3	26.6	25.8	25.1	24.5	23.8	23.2	22.6	22.0	21.4	84.1
190	58.1	55.8	53.5	51.5	49.5	47.7	45.9	44.3	42.7	41.2	39.8	38.5	37.2	36.0	34.8	33.7	32.7	31.7	30.6	29.8	28.9	28.1	27.3	26.5	25.8	25.1	24.4	23.8	23.2	22.6	22.0	86.4
195	59.6	57.2	55.0	52.8	50.8	48.9	47.1	45.4	43.8	42.3	40.8	39.5	38.2	36.9	35.7	34.6	33.5	32.5	31.5	30.6	29.6	28.9	28.0	27.2	26.5	25.7	25.1	24.4	23.8	23.2	22.6	88.6
200	61.2	58.7	56.4	54.2	52.1	50.2	48.3	46.6	44.9	43.4	41.9	40.5	39.1	37.9	36.7	35.5	34.4	33.4	32.3	31.4	30.5	29.5	28.7	28.0	27.2	26.4	25.7	25.0	24.4	23.8	23.2	90.9
205	62.7	60.2	57.8	55.5	53.4	51.4	49.5	47.7	46.1	44.5	42.9	41.5	40.1	38.8	37.6	36.4	35.3	34.2	33.2	32.2	31.1	30.3	29.4	28.5	27.8	27.1	26.4	25.7	25.0	24.4	23.7	93.2
210	64.2	61.6	59.2	56.9	54.7	52.7	50.7	48.9	47.2	45.5	44.0	42.5	41.1	39.8	38.5	37.3	36.1	35.0	34.0	33.0	32.0	31.1	30.2	29.4	28.5	27.8	27.0	26.3	25.6	25.0	24.3	95.5
215	65.7	63.1	60.6	58.2	56.0	53.9	51.9	50.1	48.3	46.6	45.0	43.5	42.1	40.7	39.4	38.2	37.0	35.9	34.8	33.7	32.8	31.8	30.9	30.0	29.2	28.4	27.6	26.9	26.2	25.5	24.9	97.7
220	67.3	64.6	62.0	59.6	57.3	55.2	53.2	51.2	49.4	47.7	46.1	44.5	43.1	41.7	40.3	39.1	37.8	36.7	35.6	34.5	33.5	32.6	31.6	30.7	29.9	29.1	28.3	27.6	26.8	26.1	25.5	100.0
225	68.8	66.0	63.4	60.9	58.6	56.4	54.4	52.4	50.5	48.8	47.1	45.5	44.0	42.6	41.2	39.9	38.7	37.5	36.4	35.3	34.3	33.3	32.4	31.4	30.6	29.7	28.9	28.2	27.4	26.7	26.1	102.3
230	70.3	67.5	64.8	62.3	59.9	57.7	55.6	53.6	51.7	49.9	48.2	46.6	45.0	43.5	42.1	40.8	39.6	38.4	37.2	36.1	35.0	34.0	33.1	32.1	31.3	30.4	29.6	28.8	28.1	27.3	26.6	104.5
235	71.9	69.0	66.2	63.7	61.2	58.9	56.8	54.7	52.8	51.0	49.2	47.6	46.0	44.5	43.1	41.7	40.4	39.2	38.0	36.9	35.8	34.8	33.8	32.8	31.9	31.1	30.2	29.4	28.7	27.9	27.2	106.8
240	73.4	70.4	67.6	65.0	62.5	60.2	58.0	55.9	53.9	52.0	50.3	48.6	47.0	45.4	44.0	42.6	41.3	40.0	38.8	37.7	36.6	35.5	34.5	33.5	32.6	31.7	30.9	30.1	29.3	28.5	27.8	109.1
245	74.9	71.9	69.0	66.4	63.8	61.5	59.2	57.1	55.0	53.1	51.3	49.6	47.9	46.4	44.9	43.5	42.1	40.9	39.6	38.5	37.3	36.3	35.2	34.2	33.3	32.4	31.5	30.7	29.9	29.1	28.4	111.4
250	76.4	73.4	70.5	67.7	65.1	62.7	60.4	58.2	56.2	54.2	52.4	50.6	48.9	47.3	45.8	44.4	43.0	41.7	40.4	39.2	38.1	37.0	35.9	34.9	34.0	33.1	32.2	31.3	30.5	29.7	29.0	113.6
m	1.22	1.24	1.27	1.30	1.32	1.35	1.37	1.40	1.42	1.45	1.47	1.50	1.52	1.55	1.57	1.60	1.63	1.65	1.68	1.70	1.73	1.75	1.78	1.80	1.83	1.85	1.88	1.91	1.93	1.96	1.98	

Height in meters

Key

Obese   Overweight   Normal weight   Underweight

Adapted, by permission, from J. Morrow et al., 1995, Measurement and evaluation in human performance (Champaign, IL: Human Kinetics), 224-225.

SCIENCE UPDATE

A large study conducted at The Cooper Institute has shown that even though a person may be classified as overweight or obese according to their BMI, it doesn't mean that they are unfit or unhealthy. In fact, men who are classified as overweight or obese but are physically fit according to a treadmill test have a lower risk of death than do men who are normal weight but unfit. This means that a person's fitness level may be a better predictor of overall health than the person's weight. That's a good reason to start being physically active, regardless of your weight.[33] ∎

Energy Balance

We have talked a lot about the importance of eating a balanced diet—one that's rich in whole grains, fruits, vegetables, and low-fat and nonfat dairy foods and includes small portions of lean meat, poultry, or fish. But you need to think about another balance, too: your *energy balance*. Energy balance, or caloric balance, is what determines your weight.

Figure 15.2 illustrates energy balance. Your energy balance is affected by the calories that you eat and the calories that your body burns. You can think of it as "energy in" versus "energy out." If you eat more calories than your body burns, the extra calories are stored as body fat. If you eat fewer calories (i.e., energy) than your body needs, your body takes some of your stored fat and converts it to energy. If your caloric intake (how much you eat) matches your energy expenditure (for movement, basal metabolism, and the digestion of food), your weight doesn't change.

The only sources of calories in your diet are foods and drinks that contain fat, protein, carbohydrates, or alcohol. These nutrients were not created equal, calorically speaking. A gram of fat contains nine calories; a gram of protein or carbohydrates contains only four calories. This means that you can eat over twice as many grams of protein or carbohydrates for the same energy cost as eating one gram of fat. Additionally, alcohol contains seven calories for every gram. Using this information, it's easier to see why some foods contain a lot of calories. These foods are often high in fat, the most concentrated source of calories in our diets. Other foods, such as vegetables, are low in fat and calories.

But just because a food is high in carbohydrates or protein and low in fat doesn't mean that you can eat as much as you want without thinking about the energy cost. You can upset your body's energy balance if you eat a lot of calories

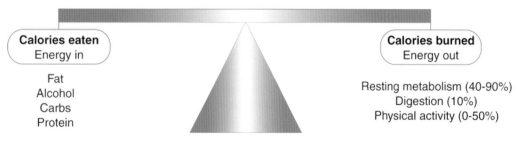

Figure 15.2   Energy balance.

no matter how high or low in fat they are. You probably know people who are eating low-fat and fat-free foods and gaining weight. How can this be? It's because they are forgetting that fat-modified foods still have calories! In fact, extra sugar is added to many fat-modified foods to compensate for the loss of flavor caused by the fat removal. If you're trying to lose weight, you can't eat all you want of a low-fat or fat-free food. Low-fat foods are not always a calorie bargain. Reading the food labels will help you make better choices.

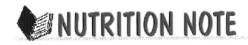

PORTION DISTORTION

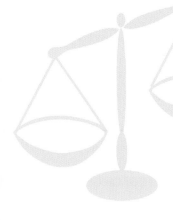

Do you sometimes eat a large portion of a low-fat food because it's low-fat? A recent study conducted in Denmark showed that subjects who chose low-fat foods ate and drank significantly more than did subjects who chose higher-fat foods. Both groups ate almost the same amount of calories and fat regardless of their food choices. The researchers concluded that larger portion sizes of low-fat foods may be causing overconsumption and a higher overall energy intake.[34] So even if you make the good choice of a low-fat food, be careful about how much of it you eat.

Although you control how many calories you put into your body each day, your body controls some of the total energy it uses. Beating your heart, moving your lungs, and maintaining your body temperature all require energy. Thankfully, your body does these things without you having to think about it. *Resting metabolism* can account for 40% to 90% of your total daily energy needs. When you put food in your mouth, the digestion process kicks in automatically and may total about 10% of your daily calories burned.

The only part of your daily energy expenditure that you can really control is—that's right, your physical activity! And the amount you can burn is totally up to you. It could be as little as 0% if you stayed in bed all day or as much as 50% if you are very active. The bottom line is that if you find ways to be physically active throughout your day, you'll increase your total energy expenditure.

To manage your weight you have to keep an eye on both your caloric intake and your physical activity. And think about this: You can restrict your calories only so much because you need the nutrients that foods provide. Yet, in theory, you can do an unlimited amount of physical activity. As you can see, being active is as important as, if not more important than, diet in controlling your weight.

NUTRITION NOTE

Calories In, Calories Out

You've learned about balancing calories eaten and calories burned. Let's look at some examples of foods and various activities. Following is a list of commonly eaten foods with their caloric density and various activities performed. Guess the amount of time you'd have to perform the activity to burn the number of calories in the food. See the example provided. The answers appear on page 170.

Food consumed	Activity performed
	(based on a 150-lb or 68-kg person)
1 cup (240 ml) of spaghetti (no sauce): 200 calories	21 minutes jumping rope
1/4 pound (115 g) cheeseburger: 540 calories	___ minutes cross-country skiing (at a moderate intensity)
Medium baked potato (plain): 220 calories	___ minutes mowing the lawn
1 cup (240 ml) of broccoli: 25 calories	___ minutes running (10 minutes per mile or 6 minutes per kilometer)
1 cup (240 ml) of regular vanilla ice cream: 304 calories	___ minutes painting
12 ounces (360 ml) of regular soda: 146 calories	___ minutes playing table tennis
Medium order of fast food french fries: 360 calories	___ minutes raking leaves

If you want to control your weight, you need to focus on both sides of the energy balance equation. The energy, or calories, that you take in should be balanced with the energy, or calories, that you burn during the day. Not only do you need to know the caloric cost of the foods you're eating, but you also need to be aware of the amount of physical activity you're doing. Together, these factors play an integral role in controlling your weight.

Factors That Affect Weight

If you or someone you know struggles with weight control, you probably realize that other factors, such as aging and genetics, can play a role in controlling weight. Although energy balance is the key to managing weight, it's affected by many things. The human body is complex and unique. Unfortunately, our bodies don't always react to food and exercise in a predictable way. Some people can eat hundreds of calories without gaining weight, while others can measure out exact portions of food and still gain weight. Let's explore some reasons for this phenomenon.

- **Genetics**—Just as your eye and hair color is determined before you're born, scientists have shown that a person's weight may be affected by his or her genetic makeup. You can see this by looking at family photos or observing families around you. Children often have similar body shapes as their parents, grandparents, or siblings. Is this a coincidence? No, it's genetics! Now, before you start blaming your parents for your extra weight, remember that genetics doesn't explain everything about your weight. Your food and physical activity choices play a huge role in determining your weight, whether or not you have a family history of obesity. If you have a family history of obesity, you'll probably have to work harder than others do to maintain a healthy weight. The

Answers to Calories In, Calories Out Activity

Food consumed	Activity performed
	(based on a 150-lb or 68-kg person)
1 cup (240 ml) of spaghetti (no sauce): 200 calories	21 minutes jumping rope
1/4 pound (115 g) cheeseburger: 540 calories	58 minutes cross-country skiing (at a moderate intensity)
Medium baked potato (plain): 220 calories	34 minutes mowing the lawn
1 cup (240 ml) of broccoli: 25 calories	2 minutes running
	(10 minutes per mile or 6 minutes per kilometer)
1 cup (240 ml) of regular vanilla ice cream: 304 calories	58 minutes painting
12 ounces (360 ml) of regular soda: 146 calories	31 minutes playing table tennis
Medium order of fast food french fries: 360 calories	77 minutes raking leaves

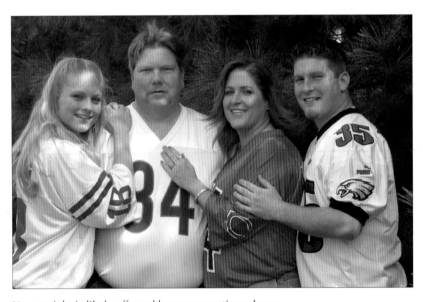

Your weight is likely affected by your genetic makeup.

skills you're learning, such as balancing calories with physical activity, watching portion sizes, and controlling triggers to eating, are especially important for managing your weight.

• **Metabolism**—Metabolism refers to the chemical processes that occur within your body that are necessary to maintain life. Your resting metabolism includes such life processes as breathing, maintaining warmth, and keeping your heart beating. Several factors affect your metabolism. These include genetics, aging, stress, illnesses, and body composition. It's become popular to use metabolism as an excuse for why managing weight is so difficult. It's true that as you age your metabolism tends to slow, but this doesn't have to result in weight changes. You can increase your physical activity or slightly reduce your food intake. This will help to combat these small changes in metabolism. Stress or illness can also result in changes to your metabolism, either increasing or decreasing your energy needs. Losing or gaining muscle mass can also affect your resting metabolism. Typically, a 180-pound (82-kg) person with more muscle mass will need more energy to maintain his or her weight than will a 180-pound (82-kg) person with less muscle mass. This means that the person with more muscle mass can likely eat more without gaining weight. Increasing your physical activity and incorporating weight training can help you boost your metabolism, especially as you age.

• **Aging**—Aging is a natural part of life. But gaining weight as we age doesn't have to be inevitable. As you age, it seems as if the weight just comes on and stays on a little easier. Why is this? First, as people age, their body composition and metabolism change. Second, people tend to do less activity as they age because of health reasons. As you age, pay attention to your body's needs. If you notice weight gains or changes in your energy level, you should adjust how much you eat or your physical activity level to balance the changes in your body. You should also be realistic in your goals. Although your body won't look like it did 20 years ago, your overall health doesn't have to suffer. Remember, health is much more than a number on a scale!

• **Emotional eating**—Many people use food as an outlet for stressors in their lives. This is called *emotional eating*. In session 5 we discussed the different characteristics of psychological and physiological hunger. Eating when you're not hungry or because you "just feel like eating" often lead to eating too many calories. This can quickly turn into weight gain, especially if you don't compensate for these calories during the day. If you are an emotional eater, review some of the ways to tackle eating triggers such as surfing the urge and planning ahead for high-risk situations.

Genetics, metabolism, aging, and emotional eating are just a few of the factors that can affect your weight. Although balancing energy is at the core of controlling weight, you should consider these other factors as you try to achieve your weight management goals.

UP CLOSE AND PERSONAL

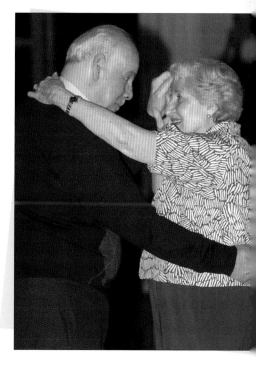

Peggy just attended her 50-year high school reunion. Her favorite local band played at the party. An avid dancer in her 40s and 50s, she was excited to get back on the dance floor. Since her husband's death 10 years ago, she'd been dancing only twice. To her surprise, she still had her dance moves, but she no longer had the stamina to dance for more than a few minutes at a time. Gone were the days of dancing through five songs without skipping a beat.

Peggy had a great time, but after the party she realized that she needed to make some changes. She wasn't sure if it was the extra weight, her lack of activity during the past 10 years, or her love of creamy desserts that was holding her back. With her best friend, Lois, Peggy decided to make a change. They registered for a weekly dance class and began taking advantage of the weekly dances at the community center. They also cut back on high-calorie desserts, and they started to eat more fruits and vegetables. Over the next six months, they both noticed changes to their bodies. They both felt as if they had more energy. Peggy began to fit into her old clothes again. She could tell that she was more physically fit and healthier overall. ▋

Controlling Weight Successfully

Throughout *Healthy Eating Every Day*, you've learned several principles that have been applied to improving your eating habits. These same strategies can be used to gain control over your weight. In fact, most successful weight-loss programs build these strategies into their programs to help their participants meet their weight-loss goals.

The most important part of a successful weight-loss program is accountability. It's easier to make and maintain changes when someone is "watching over your shoulder." That's why so many programs include weighing in at a program's office or meeting in a group setting. Recording your food intake is emphasized in many weight-loss programs. Self-monitoring helps you see what you are really eating and the amount of calories you are getting. Many programs include goal setting because it requires you to make a commitment to doing things differently. Developing your support network is important because rarely can we change without some help from others. Successful programs also teach you the importance of portion sizes and energy balance. These strategies should sound familiar because they are all essential parts of HEED, too!

Although weight loss is not a primary goal of HEED, all of the HEED goals are basic principles of losing or maintaining weight over time. By decreasing fat in your diet you will likely reduce your caloric intake. People who eat lots of fruits, vegetables, and whole grains seem to gain less weight than do people who eat low amounts of these foods. New evidence suggests that eating dairy and calcium-rich foods may help people lose weight. Finally, learning to balance calories with physical activity will help you better control your weight. As you reassess your goals at the end of this session, ask yourself:

- Was my BMI higher than I think it should be?
- Does my BMI put me at risk for chronic diseases?
- Am I gaining weight steadily over time?
- Am I ready to increase my physical activity level?

If you answered yes to these questions, you might consider focusing on balancing calories for the remaining sessions.

SCIENCE UPDATE

The National Weight Control Registry (NWCR) is a study of U.S. men and women who have successfully lost more than 30 pounds (13.6 kg) and have maintained the weight loss for at least one year. Research from the NWCR shows that balancing calories with physical activity works for weight loss and weight maintenance. In the study, 89% of the sample reported modifying *both* their dietary intake and their physical activity in order to lose weight. Only 10% used dietary modification alone, and only 1% used physical activity alone. In addition to weight loss, 85% of the participants reported improvements in energy level, self-confidence, physical health, and general mood. These results show that balancing calories with physical activity may be good for your physical *and* emotional health.[35] ▌

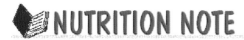

NUTRITION NOTE

Revisiting My HEED Goals

In session 10, you set short- and long-term goals for yourself. Take time now to review those goals and see if you're taking steps to reach them. How are you doing? Have you met your goals? If so, did you reward yourself appropriately?

If you weren't able to meet one or more of your goals, you should reevaluate them. In session 3, you learned about the core elements of a good goal. Remember, a goal should be personal, realistic, specific, and measurable. Look back at your goals to see if they have these core elements. A large part of goal setting is trial and error. Don't be afraid to revise your goals if you realize that they're unrealistic.

As you're reviewing your goals that you set in session 10, think about the changes you've made and the changes you'd like to make in the next few weeks. Maybe your primary goal area won't change, but you might want to revise your goals within that area or set new goals for the coming weeks. If so, use the space provided to record your new goals and rewards. You might also want to look at your HEED assessment in session 10 to see which areas of your diet you should focus on.

My Long-Term Goals (one month or longer)

Example: Within three months, I will be consistently getting 30 minutes of physical activity at least five days a week by taking the stairs at work, taking short five-minute walks during my breaks, and walking during television commercial breaks, as confirmed by reviewing notes in my daily food log.

Goal 1: _____

_____

Reward: _____

Goal 2: _____

_____

Reward: _____

My Short-Term Goals (less than one month)

Example: By next Friday, I will have reduced the time I spend sitting at home by walking the dog, cleaning the house while watching television, and walking while talking on the phone, as confirmed by notes in my daily food log.

(continued)

(continued)

Goal 1: _____

_____

Reward: _____

Goal 2: _____

_____

Reward: _____

Goal 3: _____

_____

Reward: _____

Goal 4: _____

_____

Reward: _____

Session Checklist

Before you move on to the next session's activities, be sure to do the following:

■ Complete the Finding My Body Mass Index worksheet.

■ Complete the Calories In, Calories Out worksheet.

■ Reassess your HEED goals.

■ Complete the Daily Food Log on a daily basis.

■ Visit HEED Online to learn more about weight control.

As we have discussed, controlling your weight is a matter of balancing how much you eat (your caloric intake) with your total daily energy expenditure through metabolism, digestion, and physical activity. But in real life, it's not that simple, is it? Many things, including your age, metabolism, and genes, affect your weight. Most important, though, are your daily eating and exercise habits. You can't change your age or genetics, but you can manage your weight by eating healthy foods and being physically active. You are learning many important skills that will help you adopt and maintain these habits well into the future. In session 16, you will learn strategies to keep the pressures of time and stress from wrecking your healthy eating efforts.

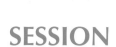

SESSION **SIXTEEN**

Managing Time and Stress

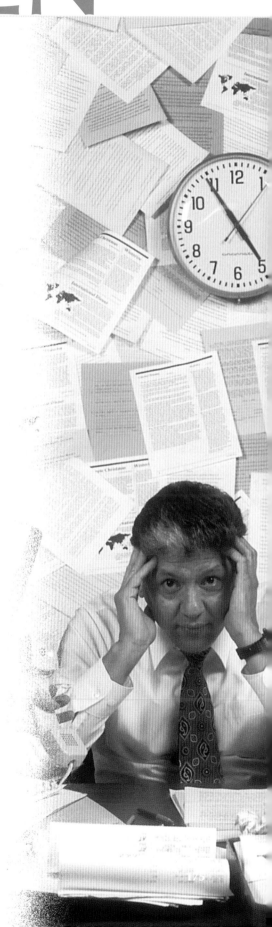

In This Session

- Identifying personal values
- Learning to act on priorities
- Understanding how stress affects eating

Much of our stress today comes from not having time to do all we need or want to do. No matter how much we would like it to be different, there will always be only 24 hours in a day. Although healthy eating doesn't have to take a lot of time, learning new healthy habits can take extra time at first. This session will help you learn to manage your time. We'll first help you set priorities, and then we'll guide you in planning ahead and getting organized. We will also review how stress can affect your eating and how diet may affect your stress level.

Managing Your Time to Help Healthy Eating Fit

Matching the activities you do with the values and priorities you believe in will help you manage your time and reduce stress in your life. Identifying healthy eating as a priority and making time to plan and organize for it can also reduce stress. In this section we'll guide you through a three-step process with three Nutrition Notes. These Nutrition Notes will help you

- identify your values and priorities,
- assess the way you spend your time, and
- plan and organize so that you are prepared to do the tasks you've set out to do.

In the end, we hope that this process fulfills two purposes: managing your time and helping you organize your life so that healthy eating fits in without causing stress.

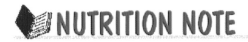

NUTRITION NOTE

Step One: Identify My Values and Priorities

The first step in effective time management is to identify your values and priorities. A *value* is a principle or quality that is important to you or is a driving force in your life right now. What's important to each person is different. For example, some people value family and faith, others value education, and others value making money. Although eating in a healthy way and taking care of one's body are values that many people overlook, we hope you have come to appreciate them.

Your values can change depending on your life stage. You might highly value making money in your 30s and 40s but shift your values to improving health and family relations in your 50s and 60s. This is only an example. The point is that because your values can change, it's important to know what you value right now.

In the space provided, list your personal values. Try to list at least five. Then rank your values by assigning each a number, with 1 being the most important value, 2 the next most important value, and so on. An example is provided to guide you.

Example:

Value	Priority	Value	Priority
Time with family	1		
Financial security	4		
Healthy lifestyle	5		
Network of friends	6		
Spiritual life	2		
Giving back to others	3		

Did you list healthy eating or anything related to maintaining good health as one of your values? If you did, how high was it ranked? If you didn't list healthy eating, don't worry. Sometimes people know they need to change their health habits, but they don't really begin to value this until they notice some benefits (such as more energy or lower blood cholesterol). Hopefully, over time healthy eating will become a driving force in your life.

UP CLOSE AND PERSONAL

Simon didn't used to pay attention to what he ate. All through his 20s he lived on fast food, packaged frozen meals, soft drinks, and quick snacks. He was focused on launching his career and didn't see the need to spend time watching what he ate. *Besides*, he thought, *I still weigh about the same as I did when I was in high school.* By the time he was 45 Simon was married, had three children, and had put on 25 pounds (11 kg). His doctor had put him on medication for high blood cholesterol and warned him about his high risk for diabetes. Simon decided he wanted to make healthy eating a higher priority both for his own sake and for his children's sake. He enrolled in *Healthy Eating Every Day* at his church. Now healthy eating is something his whole family values. ∎

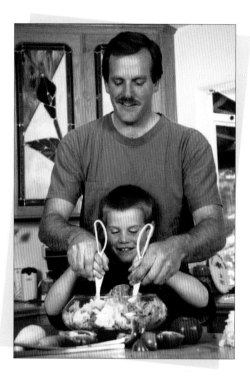

NUTRITION NOTE

Step Two: Assess the Way I Spend My Time

The next step in effective time management is to assess how you spend your time. Why? Assessing how you spend your time will show you if you are doing things you value or are actually spending a lot of time doing things that are unimportant to you. In the space provided, list all the various activities that you do and the ways you spend your time on a typical weekday and a typical weekend day. Don't labor over this task. Simply write one or two words to describe each activity. Try to include everything, big or little—working, reading the newspaper, volunteer work, cleaning your home, and so on.

Circle the items on your list that you spend the most time doing. Now review the items on your list and see if they match the values you listed in the previous Nutrition Note. Put a mark beside the activities you do that align with one or more of your values.

_____

_____

(continued)

(continued)

_____

_____

_____

_____

_____

_____

_____

_____

Did many of the activities match your values and priorities? If so, it's fair to say that you fill your time with things you feel are important and that support your values. Because you have prioritized your activities to be in line with your values, you are less likely to feel dissatisfied and stressed about the way you spend your time.

What if few activities match your values and priorities? For example, what if your faith is important to you, but you didn't list going to church, temple, or mosque among your regular activities? You may be spending a lot of your time doing things that are not important to you. This disconnect between what you value and how you spend your time can lead to feelings of dissatisfaction and stress.

Go back and review your values on page 176. What activities or strategies can you use to help you increase the amount of time you spend doing things that are important to you? Keep in mind that you may need to eliminate some of the activities you are already doing. For example, you might replace some time you spend watching TV with time spent preparing healthy meals. Write your ideas in the space provided:

_____

_____

_____

_____

Understanding your values and setting priorities are essential parts of learning to manage time better. The next step, planning, helps you make your priorities happen. Unfortunately, most people do not plan in advance how to prioritize their day. Why? It's probably because such planning takes a little extra time, at least in the beginning.

You're reading this book because you want to improve your eating habits. Presumably, healthy eating is now a priority in your life. In a moment, you are going to fill out a worksheet that will help you plan ways to make healthier choices. The task will seem a little tedious, but we guarantee that if you do it, you will be more likely to succeed in achieving your healthy eating goals. Over time, as healthy eating and being active become habits for you, you will be able to do the planning in less time and in your head.

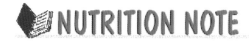

Step Three: Plan and Organize

Look at the one-day example in the following table. Notice how the person listed all of her activities for the day in the first column. Then in the second column she listed how she could incorporate healthy eating and physical activity into those tasks. Finally, in the third column she listed what she needed to do to organize for the activities and also created a shopping list (fourth column).

Activities	Healthy eating and activity strategies	Getting organized	Shopping list:
Example for one day:			Whole-grain cereal
Morning			
Serve breakfast	Serve cereal, milk, orange juice	Put walking shoes in car	Low-fat milk
			Orange juice
Drive kids to school	Walk at school track after dropping off kids		Raisins
			Low-fat yogurt
Run errands	Pack dried fruit for morning snack		Lettuce
			Tomato
Noon			Cucumber
Meet Sara for lunch	Choose large salad with grilled chicken; dressing on the side	Ask Sara to meet at restaurant with healthy choices	Carrots
			Taco shells
Afternoon			95% lean ground beef
Go to dentist appointment	Park far away from dentist's office	Get to appointment a little early	Taco seasoning
Take Jenna to piano lesson	Pack low-fat yogurt for snack with Jenna		Shredded low-fat cheese
Pick up Beth from the Joraks'			
Evening			
Make dinner	Serve tacos with lean ground beef, cheese, salsa, salad, canned peaches, low-fat milk		Peaches canned in fruit juice
Review kids' homework			Low-fat popcorn
Watch TV	Get up during commercials and march in place; snack on *one* serving of popcorn	Get out measuring utensils to measure one serving of popcorn	

(continued)

(continued)

Now it's your turn! Think about all the responsibilities, tasks, meetings, and other commitments you have for one day next week and when you will be doing them. List them in the first column of the blank table. In the second column, list specific ways that you can incorporate healthy eating and physical activity into the activities of each day. Try to be specific about the healthy eating choices you could make at each meal or snack time. Remember to keep your HEED goals in mind. This can be a good time to add any physical activity strategies.

You can't be successful with the healthy eating and activity strategies if you don't organize around your plan. In the third column, list ways that you can ensure you will be successful with your plans. Making a shopping list is a great way to make sure you have the foods on hand that are needed to put your healthy eating plans into action.

Now put your plan into action during the next week. Try to notice how planning ahead takes away some of the usual time pressure of your days.

Activities	Healthy eating and activity strategies	Getting organized	Shopping list:

Getting a handle on managing your time by identifying values, self-assessing, planning, and organizing fits nicely with other skills you have learned—namely, goal setting and self-monitoring. In terms of managing your time for healthy eating, you might want to look back at the medley of timesaving strategies for healthy cooking in session 12. In addition, you can find quick and easy recipes online and in cookbooks. Some Web sites and cookbooks have recipes that use five ingredients or less!

Time Tamers

Time management experts offer many suggestions for maximizing the limited resource of time. Here are a few for you to try:

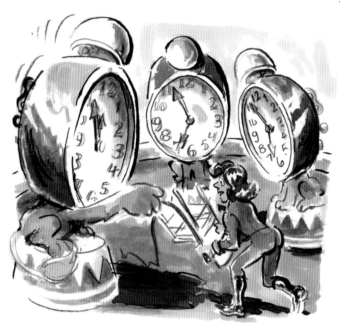

Keep a calendar. Keeping a calendar can help you keep track of all your tasks and activities, and it can keep you from overcommitting yourself. You can also look back over your calendar to see if the way you spent your time was in line with your values, goals, and plans. Calendars come in all kinds of formats, from pocket models to desk versions to handheld personal digital assistants (PDAs). Find one that works for you and your lifestyle.

Be assertive. This strategy is difficult for many people. Most of us don't want to disappoint others or appear to not be a team player by saying no. You might find it easier to assert yourself if you try to help find a solution to the request.

For example, "I greatly appreciate your asking me to help with the school committee. I'm not able to do it at this time, but I will recommend several other people who would do an excellent job." Remember, you can more easily decide whether to accept a new request for your time if you have clear values and goals.

Do "twofers." We have become a world of multitaskers. This is

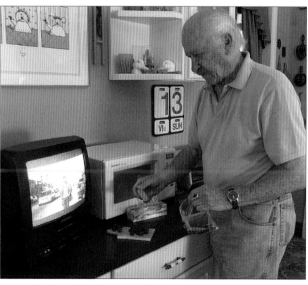

To help save time, try doing a "twofer": Pack a healthy lunch while watching television.

not always a good thing. Take driving a car and talking on a cell phone, for example. But sometimes you can do two things at one time—a twofer—that will help you lead a healthier life. For example, you can put a small television in your kitchen so that you can enjoy your favorite shows while packing healthy lunches. Walk around your child's soccer field or basketball court during practice instead of sitting and chatting with the other parents.

Delegate, delegate, delegate. You don't have to do everything! At home, in the community, and at work, recruit others to help you. Ask them to help with tasks that either are not the best use of your talents or give others opportunities to learn new skills.

Master your paperwork. Dealing with paper—junk mail, bills, memos, reports, and the like can consume a lot of time. The best time tamer with paper is to handle each item only once. When you first get a document, act on it, refer or delegate it to someone else, file it, or throw it away. It's as simple as that.

Stress and Diet

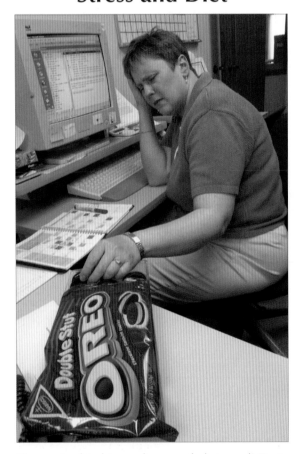

Do you tend to binge when you feel stressed? Try to calm your stress with physical activity or a relaxation strategy.

At times when you have trouble managing your time, you probably feel stressed. Understanding your values, prioritizing your tasks, and planning your activities can help lower your stress level. Eating a healthy, balanced diet can help. You'll get the energy and basic nutrients you need to combat the physical demands of day-to-day stress.

For some people, stress causes their appetite to disappear. They eat scant amounts and pay little attention to getting the basic nutrients their bodies need. If this describes you, be especially mindful about your eating habits during stressful times. Make sure that you are eating a balanced diet.

A more common problem is to use food as a way to escape or mask stressed-out feelings. Do you eat more when you feel stressed? Many people eat too much food, eat less healthy food, or both, when they are stressed. Doing so offers instant pleasure and comfort. Certain types of food may, in fact, affect mood. Some studies suggest that carbohydrate-rich foods (starches and sweets) may act as calming agents. Much more research is needed to confirm this finding. Eating as a way of coping with stress doesn't help us deal with the issue that is causing the stress. In fact, it may actually compound stress by provoking feelings of guilt, anxiety, and low self-esteem. (Remember the thoughts-emotions-behavior cycle? Look back at session 7 for a refresher.)

WEIGHTY MATTERS

Most people who are trying to manage their weight, especially during the weight-loss phase, restrict their food intake to reduce calories. These restrained eaters may be more susceptible to overeating—especially on sweet, high-fat foods—during stressful times than nondieters are. If you are trying to lose weight, it's important to learn stress management, relaxation, and coping skills that do not involve food.[36, 37]

SCIENCE UPDATE

Scientists have known for a long time that extra nutrition is needed during times when the body is under a lot of *physical* stress. For example, burn patients must undergo a tremendous amount of healing, and this requires high levels of calories and nutrients. Elite athletes whose bodies are under much physical stress also need more calories and nutrients than sedentary people do. However, researchers have not conclusively determined that people who are under a lot of *mental* or *emotional* stress need more nutrients. So don't fall for the dietary supplements that claim they will help you combat stress in your life! ▌

Stress Tamers

It's probably obvious that a high stress level is likely to negatively affect your eating habits. To stay on track with your healthy eating goals, you need to find ways to cope with stress. Here are strategies that many people find effective:

Be physically active. Physical activity is a great way to "blow off steam." The increase in body temperature, production of certain hormones, and physical exertion play a role in creating a relaxed state after exercise. Feeling good that you have done something positive for yourself can also boost your self-esteem.

Get enough rest. Sleeping restfully and getting enough sleep can help you handle the stressors in your life. Researchers recommend that you get seven to nine hours of sleep per night. Being rested can also help you maintain a positive attitude that will sustain you during stressful times.

Learn relaxation strategies. Let's face it: Stress happens. Knowing healthy ways to relax can help reduce tension and anxiety. Simple things such as deep breathing or imagining yourself in a relaxing place can be done just about anywhere and in short stints. Meditation, yoga, Pilates, tai chi, and other similar strategies may require you to learn new skills or attend classes. But they are well worth it!

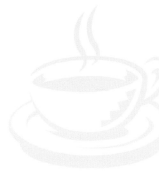

DID YOU KNOW?

Just as stress can affect your eating habits, some foods can affect your stress level. For example, excessive amounts of caffeine from beverages, medications, or other sources can cause nervousness and anxiety. This can intensify any feelings of stress and reduce your coping abilities. If you are feeling stressed, limit the amount of coffee, tea, soft drinks, and other sources of caffeine. By all means stay away from high-caffeine so-called energy drinks. They might provide a temporary boost, but they will leave you dragging after the caffeine and sugar rush has worn off.

Some people use alcohol as a way to cope with stress. Although drinking alcohol may make you feel relaxed, it's only temporary. Alcohol lowers inhibitions. You may be less mindful of making healthy eating choices when under the influence. Alcohol can disrupt your sleep pattern, which can lead to fatigue, anxiety, and additional feelings of stress. Excessive alcohol intake can increase risk of accidents, injury, and violence. Talk about adding a lot of stress to your life!

NUTRITION NOTE

Stress Eating

In stressful times, how have you used food to cope? Choose the options that best describe your actions. Review the list of strategies that you can use instead of the unhealthy options. Circle the strategies you will try the next time you are stressed out. Add any others that you think will work for you. Remember that physical activity and relaxation strategies are always healthy alternatives to stress eating.

I overate, especially on less healthy foods.

Be especially vigilant to only bring healthy foods into the house.

Call a friend when I get the urge to eat.

Be especially mindful of my portions during stressful times.

Try "surfing the urge" until the urge passes (see page 128).

Chew sugarless gum.

Keep sliced carrots, celery, and low-fat popcorn on hand to munch on when I am uptight.

Eat only in the kitchen and without other distractions, such as reading or watching TV.

Other: _____

_____

I didn't eat enough.

Have easy-to-prepare frozen meals handy.

Join family and friends at restaurants.

Have others prepare meals.

Eat on a schedule. Even if I don't feel hungry when I'm stressed, I need to refuel. Make healthy choices and use proper portions.

Other: _____

_____

I used a lot of caffeine.

Choose noncaffeinated versions of my favorite soft drinks, coffee, and tea.

Drink water instead of soft drinks.

Get plenty of sleep so that I don't need a pick-me-up.

Take frequent breaks to get up from sitting too long at my desk, watching TV, or driving a car.

Other: _____

_____

I drank a lot of alcohol.

Drink alcohol only with a meal and limit myself to one drink.

Drink nonalcoholic beverages.

Remove all alcohol from my home.

Ask family and friends to not bring alcohol into my home.

Avoid meeting friends for happy hour.

Enroll in a support program or seek professional assistance if necessary.

Other: _____

_____

We hope that by implementing some of these time- and stress-management tips, you'll feel more confident in sticking with your healthy eating plans. Even keeping to your plan will help reduce stress—you'll know that you're doing something good for yourself. The next time you feel stressed, stop and think, *Am I eating in a healthy way? Do I need to adjust how I'm spending my time? What can I do to plan and organize so that I don't feel as stressed and can still follow my healthy eating plan?*

Session Checklist

Before you move on to the next session's activities, be sure to do the following:

■ Complete the three worksheets on managing time: Identify My Values and Priorities; Assess the Way I Spend My Time; and Plan and Organize.

■ Complete the Stress Eating worksheet.

■ Complete the Daily Food Log on a daily basis.

■ Go to HEED Online to learn fun ways to manage time and stress.

If you make healthy eating a priority, you'll find it easier to make the time to shop, cook, and even eat out in healthy ways. Planning and organizing can help you focus on choosing healthy foods. Managing your time and calming your stress will help you be more successful in adopting and maintaining healthy eating habits. Learning these new skills may require some time and effort at first. But balanced eating will pay many healthy dividends down the road. In session 17, we'll celebrate your successes and introduce you to many ways to keep healthy eating fresh and fun!

SEVENTEEN

Staying Motivated

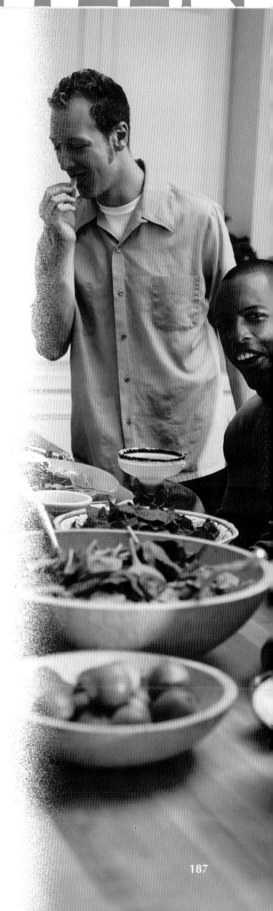

In This Session

- Celebrating successes
- Exploring new possibilities
- Beating boredom

You've made it through 16 sessions! Congratulations on following through with your commitment! When you started the journey toward healthy eating, you probably weren't completely confident that you'd get this far. But, here you are! Whether you've made drastic changes or small improvements to your eating habits, now's the time to celebrate your successes. It's time also to look ahead for ways to turn those successes into lifelong habits. In this session, we'll help you build your confidence by reviewing the changes you've made. We'll also help you avoid a "healthy eating rut" by considering ways to find new and fun opportunities for eating healthy.

UP CLOSE AND PERSONAL

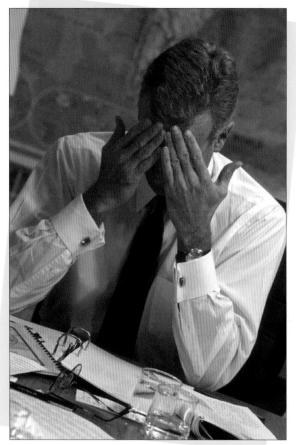

Carl is having a bad week. Not only is he behind on his daily work, but he also had a project deadline moved up two weeks. He doesn't know how he is going to have time to finish his work, much less catch up on the HEED sessions he's already behind on.

Carl originally bought the *Healthy Eating Every Day* book as part of a New Year's resolution. He was diligent for the first 10 sessions, but he has slipped a little since then. He's made a few changes—such as watching his portion sizes, learning to order more nutritious foods when eating out, and avoiding high-fat snacks—but he hasn't seen a big change in his HEED assessment scores. He sometimes wonders whether he should face the music and go back to his old ways of eating, especially now that he has new constraints on his time. Carl realizes he needs to focus on the positive. After all, he has made some very good changes in his eating habits. What can he do to keep himself going? ▮

Focusing on the Positive

Making lasting changes is not easy. Whether it's improving your eating habits, increasing your physical activity, losing weight, or quitting smoking, change occurs in steps and phases. Think back to when you started HEED. Whatever your motivation for picking up this book, you hoped that it would help you make the necessary changes to your eating habits. Just by starting HEED, you had one success. You knew you needed to make a change, and you did something about it. Since starting HEED, you've probably experienced other small victories, too.

We can measure success in many different ways. Some successes are more obvious than others. For example, if you never ate fruits or vegetables and now you eat five servings a day, you know you've been successful at meeting your goal. You may be wondering if the changes you've made are really worth the time you've spent trying to make them. The short answer to that question is *yes!* It took you years to develop your eating habits, so give yourself some time to make the adjustments necessary to cultivate a healthier way of eating. It's possible that you're overlooking some significant changes that you've already made during HEED. Let's take a few minutes to focus on the positive things that you've done over the past 16 sessions.

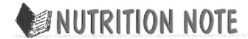

NUTRITION NOTE

Celebrating Small Successes

Review the following list of successes. Put a mark in the box next to any of the changes or accomplishments you've made up to this point. Add any additional successes at the end of the list.

☐ Started the HEED program

☐ Made improvements in my HEED pyramid assessment from session 1 to session 10

☐ Made improvements in my HEED goals assessment from session 2 to session 10

☐ Kept a daily food log much of the time

☐ Achieved one of my short- or long-term HEED goals

☐ Improved my overall health, for example, lowered my blood pressure, lowered my cholesterol, or reduced my medications

☐ Noticed improvements in my overall mood

☐ Kept up with the HEED reading materials and session activities

☐ Became a smarter grocery shopper

☐ Noticed improvements in self-esteem or confidence

☐ Tried new cooking techniques

☐ Made healthier choices when eating out

☐ Improved my ability to control my eating triggers

☐ Helped others to make changes to their eating habits

_____

_____

_____

_____

_____

Clearly, you've already made some meaningful changes during the first 16 sessions of HEED! But that doesn't mean you should stop now. If you haven't made as many changes as you'd like, there's still time. For the next few sessions, focus on meeting the goals that you set in session 15. Be sure to make healthy eating a priority in your life and plan for ways to meet your goals.

Even if you've met every goal that you've set for yourself, there are still ways to improve. The new behaviors that you've started have probably not become habits just yet. A habit is something that you value as important. You do it regardless of barriers that occur. Ultimately, your goal should be to make your new way of eating a habit that comes naturally to you. Finding new ways to eat in a healthy manner will keep healthy eating fun and exciting for you.

WEIGHTY MATTERS

When it comes to long-term weight loss, less can sometimes be more. Aiming for an incremental weight loss of 1 to 2 pounds, or 1/2 to 1 kilogram, per week improves your odds of long-term success. People who try to lose more than 2 pounds (1 kg) per week often have a very difficult time keeping the weight off. Taking small steps often leads to greater success than trying to do it all with one giant leap.

Exploring New Possibilities

You've probably heard the saying "Variety is the spice of life." When it comes to healthy eating, variety is essential. Variety not only ensures that you're getting the right nutrients, but it also staves off boredom. Having predictable snacks and meals may have worked when you were first trying to make changes. That same predictability, though, could hinder your future success. If you find yourself slipping into an eating rut, now's the time to pull yourself out by finding new ways to add variety to your eating habits.

Over the past few months, you've probably used different techniques for finding healthy eating opportunities in your community. Following are a few examples

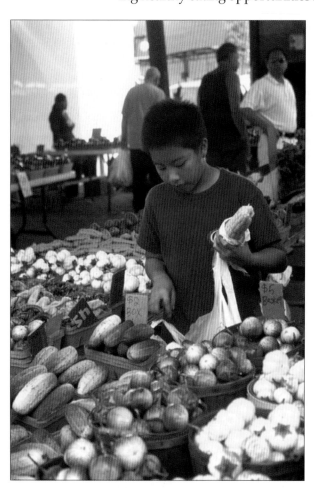

of strategies you may have used. Using one of these options can help you add to your healthy eating repertoire. Choose one strategy from the list that you haven't used before, circle it, and try to implement it during the next week. You may be surprised to see just how easy it is to stay on track while exploring new options.

- Check local papers for restaurants that serve healthy dishes.
- Ask friends and family for their favorite restaurants that have healthy options.
- Find a healthy eating friend to help you plan healthier meals.
- Share healthy recipes with family members, co-workers, and friends.
- Check the Internet for new recipes.
- Support local farmers by buying fresh fruits and vegetables at your local farmers' market.
- Join a monthly e-mail newsletter with healthy recipes and tips.
- Try new ethnic food stores for a different selection of foods.
- Subscribe to a healthy cooking magazine or buy a cookbook that has healthy recipes.

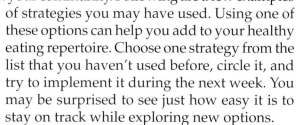

Add variety to your diet by trying a new vegetable or visiting a farmers' market.

? DID YOU KNOW?

Farmers' markets provide an opportunity for local growers to sell their own produce directly to the public. By going to a farmers' market, you'll get some of the freshest options and the best seasonal produce. You'll also get to interact with the people who actually grow the food. Many farmers' markets provide cooking demonstrations, live music, activities for children, and garden supplies. The next time you're in the mood for fresh fruits and vegetables, spend some time exploring your local farmers' market. It will be time well spent!

Cooking Up Fun

Cooking doesn't always have to be a chore. Have you ever noticed at parties that the kitchen usually turns into the social center of the party? Take a few minutes to think about the times you have enjoyed cooking in the past. Was it as a young child, helping your family prepare holiday meals? Maybe your favorite cooking times have been sharing family recipes with your own children. There are many ways to make cooking enjoyable. Here are a few ways we suggest to broaden your cooking horizons while also maintaining a healthy way of eating.

Start a healthy supper club. Ironically, as eating away from home has increased, supper clubs have become very popular. At a supper club, a group of people gathers for dinner in one location (usually one person's home), and each person brings one part of the meal. Supper clubs are a lot of fun! You can use a healthy supper club to support each others' new eating habits. Start by having a planning meeting with people who are interested in participating. Think about inviting friends, co-workers, or new healthy eating friends. At the first meeting, lay out the guidelines for the group. For example, discuss what night, how often, and where you will meet. You should also discuss menus for upcoming suppers and have everyone choose a dish to make for the meal. Remember, this is supposed to be fun, not stressful. The dishes don't have to be culinary masterpieces. They only need to be healthy options.

Be progressive. If you have neighbors who are also trying to eat healthily, you might all enjoy a progressive dinner. Progressive dinners involve eating different courses of a meal at different homes. You start with an appetizer at one home, then move to the next home for soup or salad, have a healthy main course at the third home, and finally, enjoy dessert at the last home. As with a supper club, progressive dinners provide an opportunity to support your neighbors' healthy eating habits. If you live near each other, you'll get the added bonus of some physical activity between courses by walking to each house. Start by talking to your neighbors to see who's interested in hosting a course of the meal at their house. Then plot out the best way to plan the meal.

Share cooking duties with your significant other or a friend. Sometimes being in charge of multiple meals for a week can be overwhelming for one person. No wonder so many people would rather grab a meal on the go than cook at home! There's an easy and enjoyable solution for this problem. Pick a friend, co-worker, or significant other to try this strategy with. When you're planning meals for the week, assign one person the title of "head chef" and the other

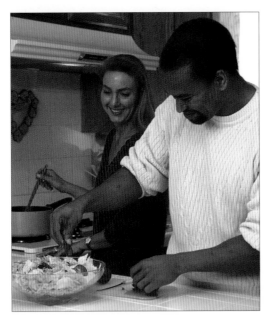
Sharing cooking duties can lighten the load.

person the role of "assistant chef" for each meal. Be sure to rotate responsibilities during the week or month. The head chef's job is to plan the meal and lead the cooking charge. The assistant chef's role is to assist with chopping, mixing, or cleaning as needed. This is a fun way to take the burden of cooking off one person's shoulders. You can also use meal preparation as a time to catch up on the day's events. To enjoy your meal even more, turn off the television and let the answering machine pick up telephone calls.

Host a theme-based dinner party. Trying new cuisines can add excitement to your new eating habits. What better environment to try a new cuisine than to have a theme party inspired by the cuisine? Dressing up doesn't have to be necessary, but it can add to the fun! First, choose a cuisine that you want to try or that you know will be popular. Ask friends or co-workers for ideas or for healthy recipes. For more ideas, you can check your local bookstore or library. Most have a large selection of cookbooks from around the world. Once you've decided on your theme and menu, send out theme-based invitations or a colorful e-mail to invite your friends to the party. Be sure to let your guests know whether they're expected to dress up or bring a theme dish for the event. Try to get decorations that fit the theme, and play music to set the tone for the party. Your guests will be so entertained that they probably won't even realize they're also eating healthy food!

Plan family dinners. Family dinners can be a great way to share your new eating habits while also sharing quality family time. At family dinners you can catch up on your children's and spouse's daily events and provide positive reinforcement. Start by setting aside one or two nights a week for a family dinner. Set family dinner times on a calendar so that all family members can work their schedules around them. Choose quick and easy recipes so that you don't spend all your time in the kitchen. By picking easy recipes, you can even give children small cooking tasks depending on their age. Try to have all family members participate, from setting the table to doing dishes. Keep the dinnertime conversation pleasant by talking about the day's events with each other and leaving unpleasant conversation until later. If your schedules won't allow for a meal eaten at home, you can plan your family meal to be taken on the road. Occasionally pack a picnic to eat at the park or after a sport practice.

❓ DID YOU KNOW?

Eating together as a family is good for more than communication and family togetherness. Compared to adolescents who don't eat with their families, adolescents who eat with their families are more likely to eat five or more servings of fruits and vegetables, to eat less fried foods, and to drink fewer soft drinks. They also have higher intakes of nutrients, including fiber, calcium, folate, iron, and vitamins B, C, and E.[38]

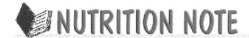 **NUTRITION NOTE**

Adding Pizzazz to Healthy Eating

Think about the ideas we have presented: starting a healthy supper club, organizing a progressive dinner, sharing cooking duties, hosting a theme-based party, and planning family dinners. Choose one of these options to implement during the next month. (If you have another idea that would work better for you, try it.) Use the worksheet here to plan the event. Keep in mind that you don't have to plan or do the event by yourself. Enlist the help of those around you. Remember that some events take more time and planning than others. If your schedule doesn't allow for a time-consuming event, pick an opportunity that fits your schedule better.

Example: Planning steps for a healthy supper club

Type of event: Start a healthy supper club

Date of event: May 15

Activities to do	People involved
Step 1: Let friends, family, and neighbors know about my plans to start the club.	*Mary, Amy, Paul, Robert, Sue*
Step 2: Organize a meeting of those interested.	*Mary, Paul, Sue*
Step 3: Decide on a night and healthy recipe assignments; volunteer to host the first supper club meeting.	*Mary, Paul, Sue*
Step 4: Remind everyone a week in advance about his or her responsibilities.	*Mary, Paul, Sue*
Step 5: Go grocery shopping and clean house.	*Me*

Additional steps or event notes: Be sure to schedule the next event or meeting at the end of the supper!

Type of event: _____

Date of event: _____

Planning activities:

Activities to do	People involved
Step 1:	
Step 2:	
Step 3:	
Step 4:	
Step 5:	

Additional steps or event notes:

⦿ PORTION DISTORTION

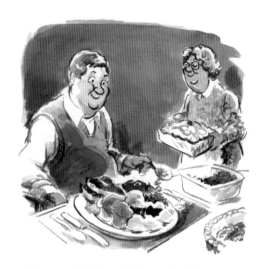

Restaurants aren't the only ones serving big portions anymore. Americans are serving themselves restaurant-sized portions at home, too. A recent study that examined U.S. national survey data from 1977 to 1998 showed that portion sizes are increasing both in restaurants and at home. This can lead to eating more calories without realizing it.[39] If you think this might be happening to you, review the serving size descriptions in sessions 1 and 7 to remind yourself of what a serving size really is.

Planning new and different ways to support your healthy eating habits may take a little time, but it will be well worth it! Be realistic for your situation: If starting a supper club is too overwhelming for you, simply invite a neighbor over for a meal. If planning several family dinners is too much to think about, plan only one to start with. The point is to mix things up a little so that healthy eating remains fresh and fun for you.

Session Checklist

Before you move on to the next session's activities, be sure to do the following:

- Complete the Celebrating Small Successes worksheet.

- Complete the Adding Pizzazz to Healthy Eating worksheet.

- Complete the Daily Food Log on a daily basis.

- Go to HEED Online for more ideas about healthy eating with friends and family.

In this session, you celebrated the important changes and successes you've experienced so far in HEED. We hope this has inspired you to continue making changes until you've developed lifelong healthy eating habits. Also, by finding new opportunities to eat in healthy ways, you've learned how to avoid getting bored with your new way of eating. You might choose to explore new restaurants or organize a progressive dinner in your neighborhood. Making healthy eating more fun and including your friends and family will lead to continued success. Keep these ideas in mind as you approach the last few sessions of HEED. In session 18, we'll talk about how our food supply is changing and the impact this may have on maintaining a healthy eating pattern.

EIGHTEEN

Eating in a Changing World

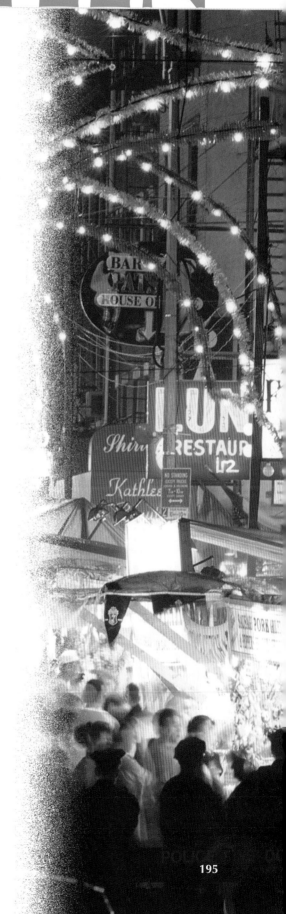

In This Session

- Understanding our toxic food environment

- Learning about vegetarianism and other alternative eating patterns

- Keeping food safe to eat

- Looking ahead to new food technologies

Change is inevitable. The nutrition world is no different. It is a very dynamic field, with many changes on the horizon. What does the future hold when it comes to food and nutrition? You may have heard news stories involving alternative eating patterns, the need to keep food safe, biotechnology, and organic foods. This session gives you a taste of the issues and trends that will likely affect our eating patterns in the years to come.

Our Food Environment

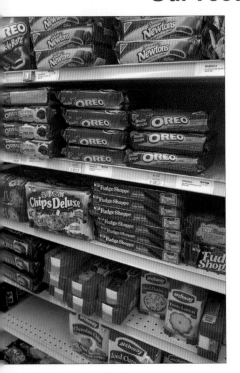

We're surrounded by unhealthy food choices.

Near our offices in Dallas, Texas, is a busy four-way intersection. There are 136 different businesses in the intersection. Consumers can buy food (and much of it not so healthy) at nearly 50 of the businesses. Not all of these are restaurants or supermarkets. We know that this isn't the only place in the world with so many food choices. Think about the community in which you live. It's likely that you don't have to go far or spend a lot of time to get something to eat.

The ease and convenience of getting food, especially foods and beverages that have low nutrient value (foods at the top of the HEED pyramid), have prompted some health professionals to warn that we are living in a "toxic food environment"—not toxic in terms of being poisonous, but toxic meaning excessive and ever-present amounts of foods that don't promote good health. Living in this kind of environment makes it difficult for people to make healthy food choices on a regular basis. This constant bombardment of food, coupled with our lack of exercise, leaves little doubt why overweight and obesity rates are continuing to climb in most Western countries.

You don't have to let the toxic food environment destroy your healthy eating efforts. The skills that you have learned in HEED have prepared you to not only survive, but to thrive, in an unfriendly food environment. The rest of this session addresses other nutrition trends and topics that may play a role in the way you eat and the foods you choose in the future.

? DID YOU KNOW?

Nabisco first introduced the Oreo cookie in 1912. In 1975, Double Stuf Oreos were introduced. Since then, Nabisco has created 10 other Oreo styles, such as fudge-covered, chocolate creme, peanut butter and chocolate creme, and the like. In addition, in the United States, you can buy seasonal varieties (Halloween with orange filling, Holiday with red filling), mini bite size and football-shaped Oreos, and Oreo candy bars. This is an example of a food manufacturer developing a strong brand and then capitalizing on the brand name to sell new versions of the product. Did consumers ask for all these different kinds of Oreo cookies? No. Nabisco created new versions and used extensive marketing and advertising to convince consumers they wanted them.

Food Trends

Food fads come and go. But here are several trends that are here to stay and will likely pick up steam in the years ahead.

Convenience is king. Today's and tomorrow's harried consumers will devour just about any quick cuisine that food companies can create. We frequently choose meal replacements bars and shakes and ready-to-eat, grab-and-go, heat-and-eat, and mobile meals. Next to taste, convenience is the most important reason people give for selecting the foods they eat.

Variety is the spice of life—and eating. Although fast food chains (e.g., McDonald's, Burger King) are holding their own, quick casual dining is gaining ground. This includes restaurants such as Chili's and Applebee's (U.S.), Kelsey's (Canada), and Frankie and Benny's (UK). People want more variety in the types and flavors of food they can enjoy. Expect to see more ethnic cuisines, new flavors, new foods (especially from countries other than your own), and new dining experiences in the years to come.

Promoting health is important. Despite what has been in the news lately, consumers continue to be concerned about the fat, sugar, and calories in foods. They want their foods to be pure, wholesome, and organic. Consumers are also turning to functional foods to prevent or treat a variety of medical conditions and ailments (see page 204 for more information). There is no end in sight for this trend.

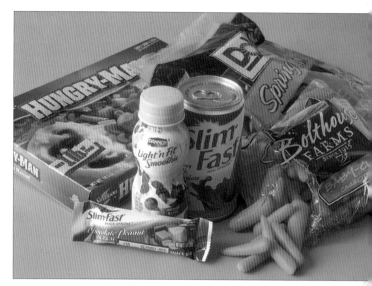

The trend of prepackaged convenience foods is here to stay.

The Vegetarian Trend

Vegetarians are not yet a big proportion of most countries' populations. But there is growing interest in this style of eating. People choose to become vegetarians for many reasons. Some, such as Seventh-Day Adventists, do it for religious reasons. Others believe that killing animals is cruel and unethical. Still others choose vegetarianism to spare the environment. The argument is that it takes many resources (soil, water, fuel, and grain) to feed the animals that then become food for humans in the form of meat and poultry. Eating low on the food chain, as vegetarians do, saves these valuable resources.

Many people adopt a vegetarian diet because of the potential health benefits. Studies have shown that people who eat well-balanced vegetarian diets have lower risks of obesity, heart disease, diabetes, and some cancers. They also tend to live longer than people who eat meat.

There are several different types of vegetarian diets:

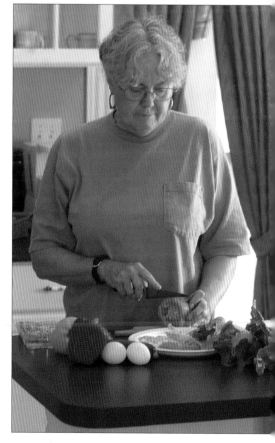

Eating the vegetarian way can be good for you.

- **Vegan**—Eats only plant foods (e.g., legumes, vegetables, fruits, grains, and nuts); does not eat *any* animal products.
- **Lacto-vegetarian**—Will eat milk, cheese, and yogurt in addition to plant foods.
- **Ovo-vegetarian**—Will eat eggs in addition to plant foods.
- **Lacto-ovo-vegetarian**—Will eat dairy products and eggs in addition to plant foods.
- **Partial vegetarian**—Plant foods provide the basis of the diet. Will very rarely eat meat, poultry, or fish, or will restrict intake to one type (e.g., only fish or only poultry). People who follow such a diet could also be called *flexitarians*.

All of these eating patterns can be healthy and well-balanced. Because animal foods are good sources of vitamins B_{12} and D, iron, zinc, and calcium, vegans (who have the most restrictive diet of all vegetarians) have to be especially mindful of their food choices. Vegans and other vegetarians can make sure they're getting the nutrients they need by including a variety of fortified whole-grain breakfast cereals, fortified soy milk, legumes, nuts, dark green leafy vegetables, calcium-fortified orange juice, and whole-grain breads in their diets. Taking a multivitamin with 100% of the Recommended Dietary Allowance (RDA) for each of these nutrients will also help.

Most vegetarians are lacto-ovo and partial vegetarians. These vegetarian eating styles are the most likely to provide adequate amounts of nutrients and

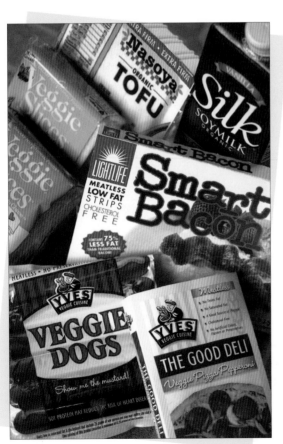

calories. By choosing low-fat or nonfat dairy products and primarily eating egg whites instead of whole eggs, the vegetarian styles can be very heart healthy. Partial vegetarians who choose to include fish in their diets also benefit from the healthy fats that are found in many types of fish.

Have you ever considered a vegetarian lifestyle but wondered if you'd get enough protein in your diet? It's true that foods that come from animals—for example, meat, poultry, fish, and dairy foods—are good sources of protein. They provide all the protein building blocks (called *amino acids*) in the quantities your body needs. Plant foods, except for soybeans and soy products, are low in one or more amino acids. But you can get enough of all the important amino acids by eating a variety of plant foods such as whole grains, cereals, legumes, and vegetables.

The following is an example of the foods a lacto-ovo vegetarian might eat in a day.

Breakfast	**Lunch**
Ready-to-eat cereal	Lentil soup
Low-fat milk (or calcium-fortified soy milk)	Soy burger
	Whole-grain bread
Calcium-fortified orange juice	Broccoli

Dinner   **Snacks**

Spinach salad   Almonds

Chopped egg   Raisins

Low-fat cheese   Yogurt

Apple

Low-fat milk

As you have read this section on vegetarianism, it may have occurred to you that many of the principles underlying a healthy lacto-ovo vegetarian diet are similar to what you have learned in HEED. It's true that HEED is a plant-based eating pattern. But you don't have to be a vegetarian to succeed in HEED. We have tried to take the best of what science is telling us about eating patterns that promote health. Moderate amounts of lean meats, poultry, and fish can be part of a healthy eating pattern. Whether you want to eat meat or not, the choice is yours.

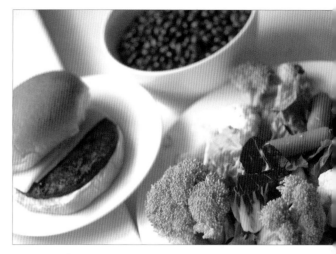

Beans, soy burgers, and vegetables are part of a vegetarian diet.

🔬 SCIENCE UPDATE

The soybean is the only plant food that provides sufficient amounts of all essential amino acids for human nutrition by itself. Eating foods made from soy is just like eating animal protein, except you don't get any cholesterol, you get very little saturated fat, and you do get some fiber. In fact, scientists have found that if you include soy in your diet you'll have lower risks of certain cancers, heart disease, and osteoporosis. Fortunately, you can find many soy-based products, such as soy milk, soy cheese, and all sorts of meat substitutes, in the marketplace. Have you ever tried a soy burger? Give it a shot. It may not taste exactly like a regular beef burger, but you just might like it—and the health benefits it provides. ▮

❓ DID YOU KNOW?

Macrobiotic Means Not So Nutritious

You may have heard about the macrobiotic eating style. It is based on the Eastern concepts of balancing yin (positive) and yang (negative). The macrobiotic diet includes multiple levels. People move from a lower level that only occasionally includes fish to upper levels that even restrict intake of fruits and vegetables! The macrobiotic style is too restrictive and may lead to nutrient deficiencies. It is not a recommended vegetarian eating pattern.

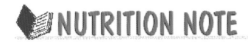 **NUTRITION NOTE**

Meatless Monday (or Tuesday, or Wednesday . . .)

Do you think you can't go a day without meat or poultry of some kind? It is easier than you think. Choose a day during the next week to go meatless. Use the space provided to write down the different foods you would likely eat. See the chart for ideas of some foods you could include. When you are done, review your menu to make sure you have included more than one food from each of the food groups in the chart.

Breakfast   **Dinner**

Lunch   **Snacks**

Possible Foods for Your Meatless Menu

Breads	Fruits and vegetables		Dairy and dairy alternatives	Meat alternatives
Whole-wheat bread	Bananas	Carrots	Low-fat milk,	Legumes
Whole-grain cereal	Pears	Spinach	yogurt, or cheese	Soy-based meat
Oatmeal	Apples	Broccoli	Soy milk, yogurt,	substitutes
Brown rice	Grapes	Tomatoes	or cheese	Eggs
Corn	Oranges	Cauliflower		Nuts
	Strawberries			

❓ DID YOU KNOW?

About 50% of the land, 80% of the fresh water, and 17% of the oil and gas used in the United States is used for the production of food.[40] Producing about two pounds (1 kg) of meat or poultry protein requires about 100 times more water than producing the same amount of protein from grains does.[41] The grain that is used to feed cows, pigs, sheep, chickens, turkey, and other livestock each year could feed over 800 million people who follow a plant-based diet.[42] Less than 3% of Americans eat a plant-based diet.[43] If more would do so, we could take great steps toward saving many of our natural resources . . . and our health.

Other Alternative Eating Patterns

Recently, other alternative styles of eating have been in the news. The **Mediterranean diet** comes from research into the diet and health status of men and women living in southern Italy, Spain, France, Greece, and Crete. People in this region tend to have lower rates of heart disease and cancer than those of people who live in other Western countries. Research now suggests that the diet eaten in this region contributes to the population's good health. The Mediterranean diet is rich in fruits, vegetables, whole-grain bread and cereals, beans, nuts, and seeds. It has moderate amounts of dairy, fish, and poultry but includes only a little red meat. The Mediterranean diet includes quite a bit of olive oil, an unsaturated fat. This finding and that of other recent research is one reason we separate out the "good" fats in the HEED pyramid. Other lifestyle habits common in the Mediterranean region, such as regular exercise and moderate intake of wine, may also positively influence health.

Have you heard about the **restricted calorie diet?** No, we don't mean the slight calorie reduction someone might follow for a few weeks or months to shed unwanted pounds. Restricted energy diets or very low calorie diets reduce caloric intake by one quarter to one half for a lifetime. Scientists have shown that rats, mice, fish, and other species who eat nutritionally adequate but low-calorie diets live longer and with lower risk of disease than do those who are fed regular diets. There are many possible reasons for this, including lower metabolic rate, lower body weight, and lower levels of hormones. Before you go cutting your calories—and food intake—in half, you should know that these results have not been confirmed in humans. Plus, given that we live in a toxic food environment, in which we are surrounded by food choices, it would be very difficult to follow such an extreme eating pattern.

Safe at the Plate

Food safety receives a good deal of attention today and is likely to receive even more attention in the future. People are concerned about how food is produced, how it is prepared at home, and how it is prepared in restaurants. Turning food into a terrorism weapon concerns some people. Let's take a closer look at these issues.

Only a small percentage of people actually produce food. For instance, in the United States, less than 3% of the population grows enough food for the remaining 97%. In addition, most countries import much of their food from outside their borders. In the United States, this accounts for millions of tons of food. Most of these raw, whole foods become ingredients in the processed foods and restaurant meals that so many of us rely on for our "grab-and-go" eating styles. The trend for less personal involvement in the growing, processing, and storing of food that began generations ago is likely to continue for many generations to come.

With all those other people involved in making your food, should you worry that what you are eating is clean, safe, and pure? The answer is no and yes. We could answer no, because many safeguards are in place to assure a safe and bountiful food supply. In fact, most Western countries have safe food systems. Still, you as a consumer should be aware of certain things to ensure that the foods you eat are clean and safe. Following are a few areas of most interest to consumers.

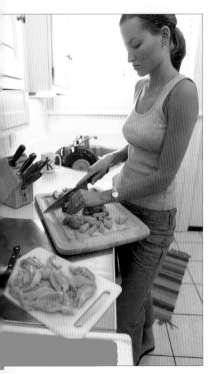

Use separate boards and knives for cutting meat, poultry, and fish.

Pesticides

Pesticides are needed to produce high yields of high-quality foods for humans and animals. But using pesticides is only one strategy that farmers use to minimize crop loss due to weeds, mold, insects, rodents, and bacteria. The use of pesticides and testing for residues are closely regulated and monitored by several government agencies to ensure compliance to established levels. To minimize health risks from contamination eat a variety of different plant foods because different pesticides are used to protect different crops. Wash all produce under clear running water. Remove outer leaves of leafy vegetables and peel produce, if possible.

Food Additives

Food additives are put in foods to preserve freshness and prevent spoilage, add or enhance flavor, add color, and aid in the manufacturing process. As with pesticides, additives are highly regulated. The Food and Drug Administration (FDA) in the United States oversees numerous layers of testing, review, approval, and monitoring to ensure that food additives are safe and used appropriately. The Food Standards Australia New Zealand (FSANZ) in Australia and New Zealand, the Food Standards Agency in the United Kingdom, and the Canadian Food Inspection Agency in Canada provide similar oversight in their respective countries. Despite popular belief, food additives have never been scientifically proven to cause hyperactivity in children.

Food-Borne Illness

Have you ever become sick from eating contaminated food? If so, you had a food-borne illness. Food-borne illness is most often the result of eating food contaminated with bacteria. The symptoms—nausea, headache, diarrhea, chills, or a fever—may mimic the flu. These symptoms usually subside in 24 to 72 hours, but severe cases can last longer and lead to long-term health problems and even death. The way food is handled, from production to storage to preparation in restaurants and at home, can influence the growth of bacteria and other illness-causing organisms. You can take many steps to minimize your risk of having your food make you sick:

- Wash your hands with warm water and soap before cooking. Also wash them frequently during cooking.
- Prevent cross-contamination by keeping cutting boards, knives, and other utensils that you use to cut raw meat, poultry, and fish separate from boards and knives used for cutting other foods.
- Use plastic or nonporous cutting boards. Wash them thoroughly in hot, soapy water.
- Never put cooked food on a plate that had raw meat, poultry, or seafood on it.
- Cook foods thoroughly and keep them hot until served.
- Use a meat thermometer to be certain that meat and poultry are cooked all the way through.

- Keep cold foods cold. Don't cram your refrigerator so full of food that the cold air cannot circulate properly.
- Refrigerate or freeze prepared foods and leftovers within two hours. Be sure to cook thoroughly when reheating.

Bioterrorism

Bioterrorism is a relatively new food safety concern. Although contamination of our food and water supply with biological or chemical agents is one way terrorists could hurt people and their countries, terrorism experts think that the risk is very slight. First, because of the great variety of foods and food producers distributed throughout most countries, it is not likely that terrorists could contaminate enough foods to affect a large part of a country's population. Thus, any attack would be relatively small and isolated. Second, as we discussed, most countries' food supplies are very closely monitored for safety. Third, if contamination were to occur, the public health system has an extensive surveillance system in place that will quickly identify an outbreak of illness, isolate the cause of illness, contain the outbreak, and implement treatment protocols. Fourth, most food companies in the United States and other countries have significantly enhanced the security measures at their manufacturing plants since the threat of terrorism became known.

The Future of Foods

It's difficult to predict what is in store for our food supply. However, several trends are sure to gain momentum in the coming years.

Biotechnology

It's hard to imagine life without frozen dinners, bagged salads, or microwave popcorn. But just 50 years ago these products weren't even on the market, much less considered household necessities. The constantly changing food market is affected not only by our taste buds, but also by technology. That's right. Improved technology doesn't only mean we'll have faster computers and better cars. It can also mean we'll have new, better-tasting foods and more of them. The advantages of food biotechnology include more efficient production of food, less spoiling, improved taste, extended shelf life of products, and improved nutrient composition. Food producers can achieve these results through modifying the genetics of plants and animals, developing improved packaging materials, and irradiating foods to eliminate contamination by microorganisms.

On the other hand, using technology has some disadvantages. Many people have concerns about scientists tampering with nature. Some people believe that altered foods are unsafe. In the United States, the FDA reports that foods produced through biotechnology aren't different from those produced conventionally.

Organic Foods

If you have concerns or ethical issues with food biotechnology, perhaps organically grown foods are the way to go for you. The organically grown food market

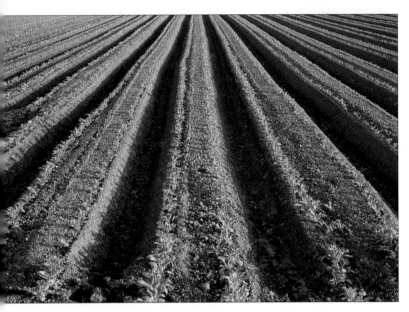

Organic foods are grown without using conventional pesticides, fertilizers, bioengineering, antibiotics, or growth hormones.

is booming. You've probably seen organically grown foods at your local supermarket. Maybe you've been tempted to take the "organic plunge." But what exactly does *organically grown* mean, and are these foods really better for you? Organically grown foods are produced without using conventional pesticides, fertilizers, bioengineering, antibiotics, or growth hormones. The United States Department of Agriculture (USDA) has established an inspection system to ensure that farmers who claim to produce organic foods are following the regulations. Look for the "USDA Organic" label on foods to tell you that a product is organic, although this label is voluntary and not used by all producers. The Australian Quarantine and Inspection Service, the Department for Environment, Food, and Rural Affairs in the United Kingdom, and the Canadian Food Inspection Agency oversee organic food production in their respective countries.

People choose organically grown foods for many reasons. Some choose these foods for various ethical reasons. Others believe organically grown foods taste better. Still others just simply like to support farmers who are looking out for the environment. Organically grown foods are usually more expensive than conventional foods are, and they don't have any additional nutritional value. The only known difference between these types of foods is how they're grown, handled, and processed. Choosing organically grown fruits and vegetables or organically produced meats and dairy products isn't as important as choosing the most nutritious foods from these food groups.

Functional Foods

You can ensure you're getting the most from the foods you're eating by consuming foods that have beneficial health effects beyond basic nutrition. These types of foods are known as *functional foods*. Some functional foods are naturally good for our health without producers adding anything to them. Other functional foods are enriched, fortified, and enhanced to provide health benefits. Oatmeal is an example of the first: It has the natural benefit of lowering people's cholesterol levels. You have probably seen foods that have extra health-enhancing ingredients added to them. For example, several margarines contain an ingredient to lower blood cholesterol levels. This ingredient doesn't naturally occur in margarine. It has been added to provide this extra benefit. Maybe you've purchased bread that has extra calcium added to it. This is another example of a functional food. Given most people's interest in improving their health and well-being, food manufacturers are searching hard for other ways to boost the nutritional value of food products by adding additional, healthy ingredients.

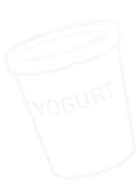 UP CLOSE AND PERSONAL

Melissa and Susan work together as aides at a local school. Both have grown children but have volunteered because they enjoy the children and the energetic atmosphere. One day Susan reported that at a recent check-up, her doctor told her she was in the early stages of osteoporosis. Susan said her doctor had recommended she do more physical activity and eat plenty of calcium-rich foods. Susan knew that dairy products were the best source of calcium. "But," she told Melissa, "I don't like the taste of many dairy products. What am I going to do?" Melissa's sister was coping with the same problem, so Melissa shared some of her sister's strategies with Susan. As often as she can, Melissa's sister eats the low-fat dairy products that she does like. She also eats functional foods that are fortified with calcium. These include certain types of soy milk, orange juice, breakfast cereals, and bread. And she takes a calcium supplement. Susan felt better knowing there were so many ways to boost her calcium intake without having to eat only dairy products. ∎

Session Checklist

Before you move on to the next session's activities, be sure to do the following:

- ■ Complete the Meatless Monday worksheet.

- ■ Complete the Daily Food Log on a daily basis.

- ■ Go to HEED Online for more information on food safety and functional foods.

In this session, we covered many emerging topics, ranging from food trends to food safety to functional foods. One of the aims of HEED is to give you information to help you make the best food choices possible to improve your overall diet quality. Use the information in this session to continue on your path to better eating. In session 19, you'll identify the strategies that have worked best for you. You'll also plan ways to get back on track if you find yourself slipping once you have completed HEED.

NINETEEN

Planning Ahead

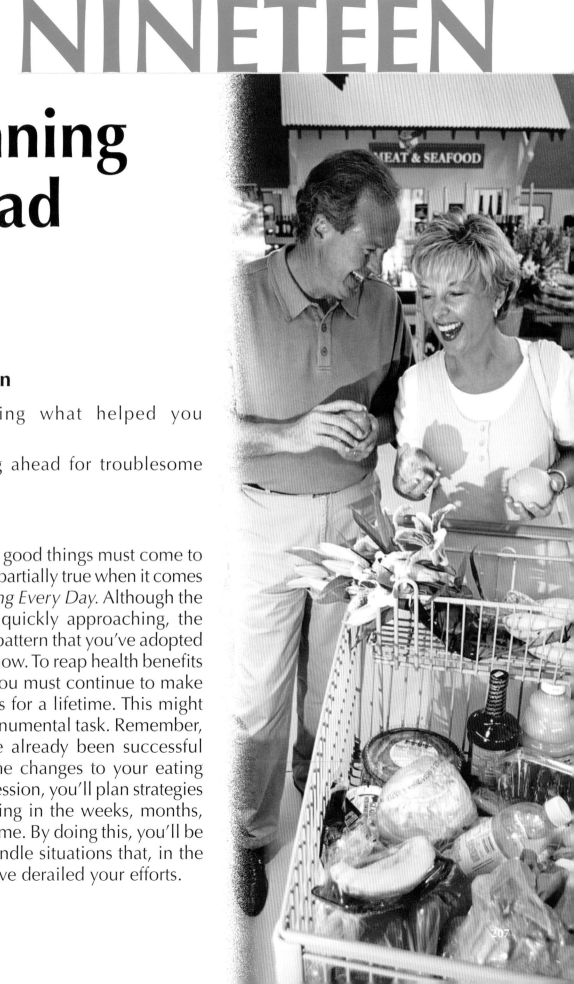

In this Session

- Identifying what helped you change
- Planning ahead for troublesome times

The saying "All good things must come to an end" is only partially true when it comes to *Healthy Eating Every Day*. Although the last session is quickly approaching, the healthy eating pattern that you've adopted shouldn't end now. To reap health benefits in the future, you must continue to make healthy choices for a lifetime. This might seem like a monumental task. Remember, though, you've already been successful in making some changes to your eating habits. In this session, you'll plan strategies for healthy eating in the weeks, months, and years to come. By doing this, you'll be prepared to handle situations that, in the past, would have derailed your efforts.

207

Taking Stock

In HEED, we've addressed many different areas in our attempt to help you make better food choices. We introduced you to the HEED pyramid (figure 19.1). The HEED pyramid emphasizes the importance of whole grains; colorful fruits and vegetables; healthy protein choices such as poultry, fish, legumes, and nuts; and low-fat and nonfat milk, yogurt, and cheese. The HEED pyramid also does something that most food guides don't do: It emphasizes the importance of daily physical activity for balancing calories and for overall health. As you continue, use the HEED pyramid as your guide for making the healthiest choices possible in each of the pyramid food groups.

We also introduced you to new ways of thinking about food and eating. Remember the phrases "All foods can fit" and "Focus on getting nutrients from whole foods"? You had several chances to track your progress: You periodically completed the HEED assessments and revisited your short- and long-term goals. Hopefully, these signposts helped you to stay on track and gave you a chance to reevaluate the direction you wanted to go. You also learned some great nutrition information: You discovered the latest information about the many benefits of a

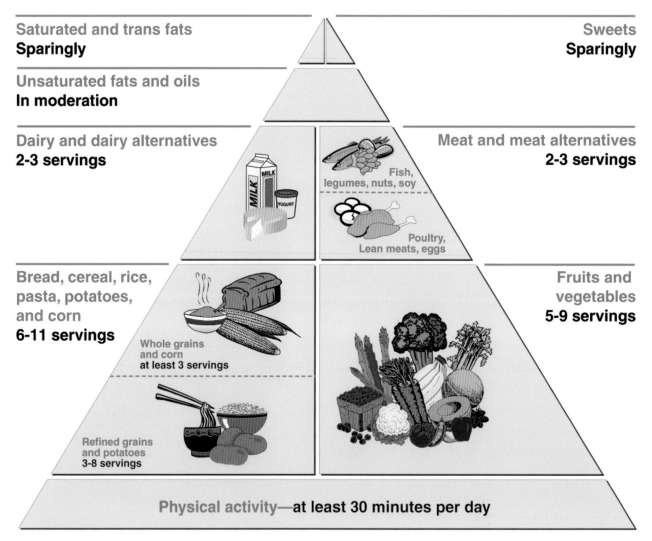

Figure 19.1 Healthy Eating Every Day pyramid and HEED goals.

healthy diet, and you learned the lowdown on supplements and fad diets. You explored how to be a smart shopper and how to eat in a changing world. You learned new skills for tracking your eating habits, preventing lapses, eating out, coping with eating triggers, and many others. We also provided you with many healthy eating resources that you could pursue on your own.

We don't expect that you used every concept, skill, or resource we've offered. It's very likely that you found some of the strategies worked better for you than others did. No set of strategies will work the same for two different people. One of the unique things about HEED is that you can tailor it to your own needs. Just as you chose areas of your diet that you wanted to work on, you should also select the strategies that work best for you.

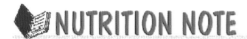

NUTRITION NOTE

What Helped Me Change

What strategies work best for you? Take a few minutes to review what you found most helpful in the process of adopting healthier eating habits. Carefully review the following list of items. We've included five categories: attitudes and philosophies, information, new skills, helpful resources, and others. Read through the entire list first. Carefully think about which approaches or strategies were the most helpful to you. If you found something particularly helpful but it's not on the list, add it under the "Others" category. After you've read through the entire list, place a mark beside the five things that were the most helpful to you.

Attitudes and Philosophies

❏ A balanced diet—that is, eating from all food groups—is important (sessions 1, 2, 3, 10)

❏ All foods can fit (preface, sessions 1, 5)

❏ Focus on getting nutrients from whole foods (sessions 1, 2, 3, 10)

❏ Gradual changes are changes you can live with (sessions 1, 2, 3, 17)

❏ Progress, not perfection, is what counts (sessions 5, 11, 17)

❏ All five HEED goal areas are important (sessions 1, 2, 3, 10, and there's more to come in session 20)

Information

❏ Understanding my stage of readiness to change (session 1)

❏ Understanding my barriers to healthy eating (session 4)

❏ Knowing benefits of healthy eating (sessions 1, 2, 4, 10, 20)

❏ Understanding the definitions of functional and organic foods (session 18)

❏ Knowing my actual dietary intake from my HEED assessments (session 1, 2, 10)

❏ Finding opportunities to be more physically active (sessions 1, 14)

❏ Balancing calories eaten with calories burned (sessions 14 and 15)

❏ Identifying ways to make healthy eating fun (session 17)

❏ Understanding dietary supplements and fad diets (sessions 13, 18)

(continued)

(continued)

◻ Identifying nutrition misinformation (session 13)

◻ Understanding alternative eating habits such as vegetarianism (session 18)

New Skills

◻ Eating proper portions (sessions 1, 3, 7, Portion Distortion segments, your daily food logs)

◻ Setting short-term and long-term goals (sessions 4, 7, 10, 15)

◻ Rewarding myself (sessions 4, 7, 10, 15)

◻ Keeping daily food logs (sessions 3 and following)

◻ Using the IDEA strategy to solve problems (session 4)

◻ Identifying new opportunities for healthy eating (sessions 4, 6, 8, 12, 17)

◻ Eating healthy when eating out (session 6)

◻ Getting support from those around me (sessions 9 and 17)

◻ Identifying and dealing with triggers for unhealthy eating (sessions 5, 7, 11, 15, 16)

◻ Preventing and coping with lapses, relapses, and collapses (sessions 5, 17, 19)

◻ Thinking positively (sessions 7, 11, 17, 19)

◻ Healthy food shopping strategies (session 8)

◻ Managing stress (sessions 5 and 16)

◻ Healthy cooking strategies and skills (sessions 12 and 17)

◻ Identifying personal values and setting priorities (session 16)

Helpful Resources

◻ HEED book

◻ HEED Online

◻ Healthy eating books, newsletters, magazines, Web sites, and other resources

Others

_____

_____

_____

_____

Take a moment to reflect on the choices that you made. Are you surprised at which items really worked for you? Perhaps it was difficult to narrow down the items to just five. On the other hand, maybe you found only one or two strategies that really worked for you. Whatever your choices were, these are the approaches that you should continue to use in the future to stay on track with your healthy eating goals. The information you have learned from HEED will tend to fade over time if you don't keep practicing the strategies that worked best. Use this What Helped Me Change worksheet to remind yourself of these strategies and where in the materials you can go to review the information in the future.

UP CLOSE AND PERSONAL

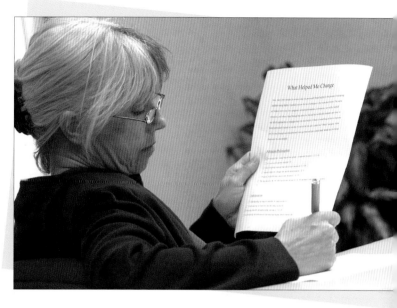

Virginia has made great progress during HEED. She's seen dramatic changes in her energy level because of the healthier choices she's making. She's also lost weight along the way. As Virginia completed the What Helped Me Change worksheet, she was really surprised by what strategies worked for her. Even though she had never written down goals for herself in the past, she found that setting short- and long- term goals really worked. Now she wishes she had picked up that skill 30 years ago! Virginia also realized that recording her daily food intake was another great way to help her stay on track. After weeks of writing down every food she'd eaten, she can now track servings of fruits, vegetables, and whole grains in her head. With every new change she's made, Virginia's become more interested in learning about nutrition. Virginia plans on maintaining her new eating habits by using these new skills and resources in the future. ▌

WEIGHTY MATTERS

For most people, losing weight and maintaining long-term weight loss are difficult. But using strategies like those introduced in HEED can help you keep the weight off. Researchers showed that people who successfully maintained their weight after having lost weight reported extensive use of behavioral strategies for reducing fat intake. For example, they modified meat preparations, avoided fried foods, and substituted low-fat foods for high-fat foods. These strategies, along with increasing physical activity, helped people to maintain long-term weight loss. Through such measures these people have improved their overall health. You can use these same approaches to make lasting changes to your eating habits.[44]

Troubleshooting

Throughout *Healthy Eating Every Day,* you have learned that lapses are to be expected. It's how you plan for and react to those lapses that determine whether you'll succeed in maintaining your new way of eating. Even though you've learned ways to prevent lapses and to tackle triggers that can lead to lapses, you should still expect lapses to occur.

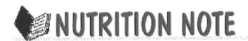

NUTRITION NOTE

My Troubleshooting Guide

You can plan for lapses by predicting some of the barriers you might face in the future. We've helped with the planning by providing a troubleshooting guide. You can use this when the going gets rough in the weeks and months to come. Listed in the left column are common triggers, barriers, and troubles that can potentially derail your healthy eating efforts. The middle and right columns list the HEED sessions and other resources that can help you overcome each particular challenge. As you're scanning the list, you may think of other triggers or challenges that you anticipate facing in the future. Add those to the bottom of the list along with potential solutions for the problem from HEED sessions or other resources.

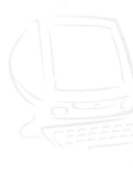

Trouble or challenge	HEED sessions	Other resources
Got off track; having trouble getting back on	3, 4, 5, 7, 9, 10, 11, 17, 19, 20	
What is a healthy eating pattern?	1, 2, 10, 13, 20	Nutrition newsletters, nutrition Web sites
Eating out strategies	6, 17	Calorie counter books, restaurant Web sites
Coping with holidays and special occasions	4, 5, 11	
Boredom with healthy eating patterns	6, 8, 12, 17	Cookbooks, nutrition magazines, cooking classes
How do I balance my calories with physical activity?	14, 15	Active Living Every Day program (www.ActiveLiving.info), Human Kinetics Web site, Human Kinetics resources
All-or-none thinking	4, 5, 7, 11, 17	
Feeling guilty about making a poor choice	7, 11	
How to get more dairy or calcium-rich foods	3, 8, appendix C	Nutrition Web sites
How to get more whole grains	3, 8, appendix C	Nutrition Web sites
How to get more fruits and vegetables	3, 8, appendix C	Nutrition Web sites
How to eat less fat	3, 8, appendix C	Low-fat cookbooks, low-fat menu items

Not enough time to eat healthy foods	4, 6, 12, 16	
Controlling my weight	14, 15	Weight management books and Web sites
Are my portions right?	1, 2, 3	Measuring tools, daily food logs
Getting support from friends and family	9, 17	Cooking clubs and classes
What to do about eating triggers	5, 7, 11, 16	
Choosing healthy foods when shopping	8, 12	Calorie counter books, supermarket advertisements
Making unhealthy choices because of stress	5, 7, 16	Meditation tapes, relaxation tapes
Don't know how to cook healthy foods	8, 12, 17	Cookbooks, magazines, cooking clubs and classes

Unfortunately, lapses happen to even the most mindful and prepared people. We hope that with the troubleshooting guide at your disposal, you feel better prepared to deal with any healthy eating stumbling blocks that arise in the future.

Session Checklist

Before you move on to the next session's activities, be sure to do the following:

- ■ Complete the What Helped Me Change worksheet.

- ■ Review the Healthy Eating Troubleshooting Guide.

- ■ Complete the Daily Food Log on a daily basis.

- ■ Go to HEED Online to learn more about staying on track.

Although the 20 sessions of HEED are nearly over, you are really just at the beginning of a lifetime of healthy eating. The philosophies, knowledge, skills, and resources that you have learned will help you maintain your healthy eating habits for the long haul. Keep the What Helped Me Change worksheet, the Troubleshooting Guide, and the entire HEED book handy so that you can easily refer to them when you hit a roadblock. Get ready for session 20! You'll assess your progress one last time and identify areas that you need to continue to work on.

TWENTY

Celebrating Success

In This Session

- Assessing the health of your diet
- Setting new goals and rewards
- Celebrating!

Congratulations on completing *Healthy Eating Every Day!* Be sure to reward yourself for working so hard and sticking with HEED. In this session, you'll check your progress one last time. You'll also set new goals and rewards that can keep you motivated beyond HEED.

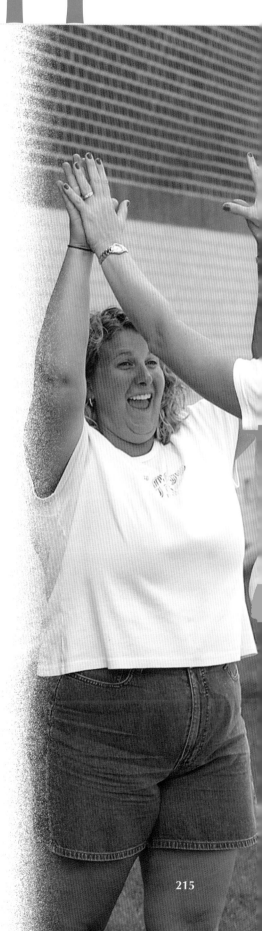

We hope that you have learned many things that will help you continue to make healthy changes in your diet. Getting health benefits from healthy eating is a lifelong endeavor. You will need to rely on the skills, strategies, and resources that you have acquired to break down barriers as they arise in the future. Let's take a closer look at your barriers and benefits.

Evaluating Barriers and Benefits

Turn to page 52 to see the list of healthy eating barriers that you cited at the beginning of HEED. Review the list of barriers carefully. How do you feel about the list today as compared to when you first filled it out? Think about why your thoughts about barriers have changed. Chances are, some of your barriers are no longer barriers because you have learned skills to get around them. Others may not seem as daunting as they did in the beginning. Cross out the barriers you listed that are no longer barriers. Have you discovered any new barriers? Add them to the list. This will help you know the areas you can continue to work on in the future.

Now review your list of personal benefits on page 50. Is this list still accurate? Have you identified any new benefits since you started HEED? If so, add them to your list. Are some benefits more important to you now than they were before?

Compare your barriers and benefits lists. Which list had more items in it in session 4? Which list has more items now? If you have been working hard to incorporate the HEED principles into your daily habits, it's likely that your benefits list now outweighs your barriers list. You also probably feel more confident and motivated to maintain your changes over time.

Assessing your barriers and benefits to healthy eating every six months can help you stay motivated for many years to come. Mark your calendar for six months from today to review your benefits and barriers list again.

HEED Goals Assessment

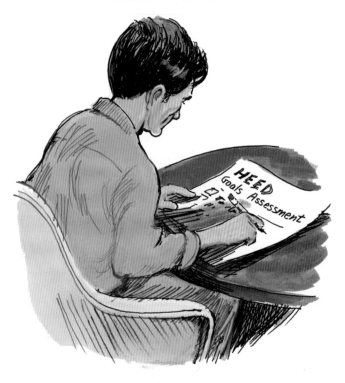

Now is a good time to see how far you have come in your efforts to make healthy dietary changes. Remember the HEED goals and HEED pyramid assessments that you completed in sessions 1 and 2 and again in session 10? In this session, you'll complete them again to evaluate your current eating habits. This will help you see what areas you can continue to work on. This should be old hat for you by this point. If you'd rather do this online, you can complete these assessments and the stages of readiness to change assessment at HEED Online (go to www.ActiveLiving.info). Let's start with the HEED goals assessment.

You completed the HEED goals assessment in session 2 and in session 10. You'll now complete it again to evaluate your current eating habits. This assessment will help you see how the quality of your diet has changed over the last 10 sessions.

Go to appendix D on page 234 to complete your HEED goals assessment. Make a copy of the assessment, and complete the HEED goals assessment by selecting one answer for each question. Read each answer carefully before choosing one. Write the score for each answer in the last column on the right. Then total the score for all questions at the bottom of each section.

Now write your scores in the HEED Assessment Log in appendix A. How do your scores compare with your scores in session 2 and session 10? In what goal areas do you now have higher scores? This indicates that you have improved in those areas. Congratulations! Are there any goal areas for which you had a lower score? Don't be discouraged. These are areas that you may wish to work on even though you've completed HEED.

Circle any items in the five HEED goal categories in which you scored a 3 or lower. These are specific areas you can focus on as you set new goals later in this session. You can retake this assessment at any time in the future to see how you are doing.

HEED Pyramid Assessment

The HEED pyramid assessment is based on the HEED pyramid (see figure 20.1). This assessment tests whether you're getting the right amount of nutrients. To get the nutrients you need, you need to eat the right number of servings from each food group. Let's see how you're doing. Complete table 20.1, My Daily Servings. You can use a day for which you have recorded your food intake on your Daily Food Log or you can estimate the servings from a typical day.

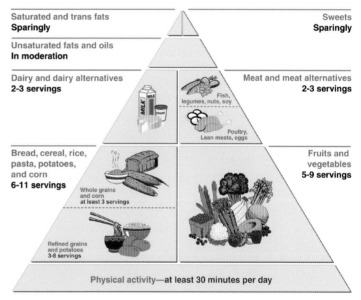

Figure 20.1 Healthy Eating Every Day (HEED) pyramid.

From *Healthy Eating Every Day,* by Ruth Ann Carpenter and Carrie E. Finley, 2005, Champaign, IL: Human Kinetics. Organizations and agencies may not photocopy any material for professional or organizational use or distribution.

1. For one day, beginning with breakfast, write down everything you eat and drink. Include breakfast, lunch, dinner, and snacks. If your eating patterns are not that different from day to day, you can simply think back over yesterday's food intake and write it in the space provided.

2. For each food you listed, identify the amount you ate or typically eat. Measure the amounts, if possible.

3. For each food you listed, identify the food group it belongs to (e.g., fruits and vegetables) and translate the quantity you ate into pyramid *servings.* (Use the Food Group Serving Sizes on page 11.) For each food you listed, write the number of pyramid servings you ate in the column under the food

Table 20.1 My Daily Servings

Meal	Food eaten	Amount eaten	Bread, cereal, rice, pasta, potatoes, and corn	Fruits and vegetables	Dairy and dairy alternatives	Meat and meat alternatives	Unsaturated fats and oils occurrences	Saturated and trans fats occurrences	Sweets occurrences
Breakfast									
Lunch									

(Servings eaten)

(continued)

Meal	Food eaten	Amount eaten	Bread, cereal, rice, pasta, potatoes, and corn	Fruits and vegetables	Dairy and dairy alternatives	Meat and meat alternatives	Servings eaten Unsaturated fats and oils occurrences	Saturated and trans fats occurrences	Sweets occurrences
Dinner									
Snacks									
Servings totals									

From *Healthy Eating Every Day*, by Ruth Ann Carpenter and Carrie E. Finley, 2005, Champaign, IL: Human Kinetics. Organizations and agencies may not photocopy any material for professional or organizational use or distribution.

group it belongs to. For instance, if you drank 6 ounces (180 ml) of orange juice at breakfast, you would write "1" under the fruits and vegetables column, because that represents one serving size of fruit.

4. Pay special attention to how to treat the two fat groups and the sweets group. There are no standard serving sizes for these groups.

- Place a 1 in the unsaturated fats and oils column for each time you eat any of the foods listed in table 1.1, Tale of Two Fat Categories, on page 9.
- Put a 1 in the saturated and trans fats category each time you eat butter, stick (hard) margarine, whole milk dairy products, fatty meats, fried foods, and the like.
- As with the fats categories, put a 1 in the sweets column every time you eat any amount of sweetened drinks, sweets, sugar, honey, cake, cookies,* pie, and sweetened desserts.

5. Finally, total the numbers in each group to view your daily intake.

How does your diet compare to what is recommended for you? Remember this step from sessions 1 and 10? Complete tables 20.2 and 20.3. First, transfer your daily intake totals to the first column in table 20.2, labeled My Daily Servings. Next, transfer your recommended servings from table 1.2, Recommended Servings for Different People, on page 12 in session 1. Then subtract what is

Table 20.2   How Does My Diet Stack Up?

Food group	My daily servings	Recommended for me	Pyramid needs
Example: Fruit and vegetable group	3	5	-2
Bread group			
Fruit and vegetable group			
Dairy group			
Meat group			

Table 20.3   Oils, Fats, and Sweets Intake

	My intake		My intake
Unsaturated oils	_____	Sweets	_____
Saturated and trans fats	– _____		
Difference	_____		

*Same as *biscuits* in some countries.

recommended for you from your actual intake. See the first row in table 20.2 for an example. This will show you whether you are eating an appropriate amount of each food group:

- If you scored zero, you are eating an appropriate amount of that food group.
- If you scored a positive number, you are eating too much of that food group.
- If you scored a negative number, you are not eating enough of that food group.

Write your total intake of unsaturated and saturated fat in table 20.3. Then subtract the saturated fat category from the unsaturated oils. Remember, you want to end up with a positive number. In other words, you want to be eating more foods that contain "good" fats than foods that contain "bad" fats.

For the sweets group, enter your total intake from the sweets column of table 20.1 in the sweets row of table 20.3. As we have said before, because these foods provide few nutrients and many calories, you want to keep this number as low as possible.

Record your results in the HEED Assessment Log in appendix A. Compare your current scores with your scores from session 1 and session 10. See figure 20.2 for an example of a completed assessment log for session 20.

Assessment 3: Session 20
HEED Goals Assessment
Date June 4

HEED goal area	HEED goals assessment score	Change from assessment 1 to assessment 2
Increasing fruits and vegetables	22	Up 1
Decreasing fats	32	Up 3
Increasing dairy products and dairy alternatives	18	Up 8 Hooray!
Increasing whole grains	18	Up 3
Balancing calories	18	Down 2
Total score	109	Up 14

HEED Pyramid Assessment
Date June 4

HEED pyramid group	HEED pyramid assessment score	Change from assessment 1 to assessment 2
Bread group	+1	No change
Fruit and vegetable group	0	Down from +1
Dairy group	0	Up from -1 Finally!
Meat group	+1	Up from 0
Fats	+4	Up from +2
Sweets	+1	No change

Figure 20.2 Example of completed assessment log for session 20.

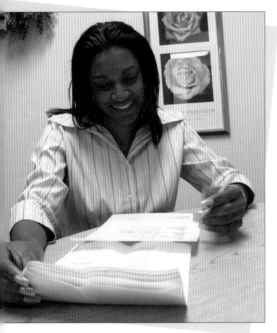

For all groups other than the fats and sugars categories, in which groups was your score a zero? This means that you are getting the right number of servings for that food group. Did you improve from a negative number to zero in any areas? If so, special congratulations to you! This means that you went from not getting enough of a specific food group to getting adequate amounts. Be careful about any food groups for which you had a number higher than zero. You may be eating more than you need for good health. Remember, even though fruits or vegetables are excellent choices, excessive amounts can add up to a lot of extra calories.

On your fats categories score comparison, if you increased your score from sessions 1 and 10, you likely have made some positive changes to decrease the unhealthy fats and excess sugars or to increase your healthy fats. Keep up the good work. If your score went down compared to your score for the earlier assessments, try to think about ways to cut down on your "bad" fats and excess sugars.

Reviewing Goals and Rewards

By now you should be a pro at setting goals and rewarding yourself! The assessments you just completed give you good information on parts of your diet that still could use some work. Take a look back at the goals and rewards you set in session 15. Have you met your long-term and short-term goals? Did you reward yourself for meeting your goals? If you had trouble meeting your goals, reevaluate the goals: Were they personal, realistic, specific, and measurable? Do you want to reset your goals using the new information from the assessments that you just completed?

Finishing HEED doesn't mean you've finished setting goals for yourself. Even if you are satisfied with your current eating habits, you can set goals for maintaining your new healthy eating skills. Take time now to set new short- and long-term goals for yourself.

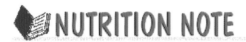 NUTRITION NOTE

Ready? Set Goals!

You've completed the HEED goals assessment and the HEED pyramid assessment for the third time. In what areas could your diet still improve? Are there goals from session 15 that you still want to work on? Do you want to change any goals based on the results of the assessments you've just completed? Take some time now to set new long-term and short-term goals.

My Long-Term Goals (one month or longer)

Example: Within three months, I will be eating less fat each day, as confirmed

by my daily food logs. I will achieve this by decreasing the amount of margarine I add to foods, by choosing fruit for dessert, and by choosing reduced-fat salad

dressing.

Goal 1: _____

_____

Reward: _____

Goal 2: _____

_____

Reward: _____

My Short-Term Goals (less than one month)

Example: By next Friday, I will have reduced the amount of fat in my diet by

substituting nonfat milk for whole milk, as confirmed by my daily food log.

Goal 1: _____

_____

Reward: _____

Goal 2: _____

_____

Reward: _____

Goal 3: _____

_____

Reward: _____

Goal 4: _____

_____

Reward: _____

It's a Wrap

In session 19 you identified the specific information, skills, and resources that you found the most helpful during HEED. You also started thinking ahead about potential barriers and ways you could overcome them. In session 20, you have identified the progress you have made and some areas that you could still improve in. In fact, we recommend you put a note in your calendar three to six months from now to complete these assessments again. This will reassure you that you haven't gradually slipped back to unhealthy eating habits.

All that is left to do is to remind you once again that the science of nutrition is very complex, but the art of eating correctly is pretty simple. Keep these simple

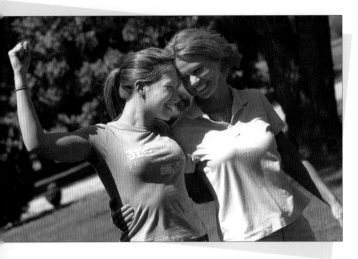

tips in mind as you work to maintain your healthy eating habits:

- Keep your HEED materials handy. If you get off track, they can help you get back on track.
- The HEED pyramid shows what a healthy, balanced daily diet should look like. Post a copy of it on your refrigerator or in another visible place as a frequent reminder to eat well.
- Maintaining a healthy eating pattern can yield significant health benefits.
- A balanced diet is best. No single food, food group, or supplement provides all the nutrients your body needs.
- All foods can fit.
- Try new foods and tastes.
- Enjoy food and eating.

Congratulations on all that you have accomplished! We wish you a lifetime of healthy eating every day.

HEED Assessment Log

The purpose of the HEED Assessment Log is for you to track your progress throughout HEED in one place. This will make it easier to see if you're making the changes you want to make. You'll complete each assessment three times: the HEED pyramid assessment in sessions 1, 10, and 20 and the HEED goals assessment in sessions 2, 10, and 20. After each assessment, insert your scores into the tables provided here. After your second assessment (session 10), compare your new scores to the scores from your first assessments (sessions 1 and 2) to see how you're doing in meeting your goals. Likewise, after your final assessment in session 20, compare your final scores to your scores from session 10. You'll be able to see areas that you've really improved in and also goal areas that you can continue to work on in the future.

Assessment 1: Sessions 1 and 2

HEED Goals Assessment

Date _____

HEED goal area	HEED goals assessment score	Readiness to change* (circle one per goal area)				
Increasing fruits and vegetables		P	C	PP	A	M
Decreasing fats		P	C	PP	A	M
Increasing dairy and dairy alternatives		P	C	PP	A	M
Increasing whole grains		P	C	PP	A	M
Balancing calories		P	C	PP	A	M
Total score						

HEED Pyramid Assessment

Date _____

HEED pyramid group	HEED pyramid assessment score
Bread group	
Fruit and vegetable group	
Dairy group	
Meat group	
Fats	
Sweets	

* P = Precontemplation; C = Contemplation; PP = Preparation; A = Action; M = Maintenance

Assessment 2: Session 10

HEED Goals Assessment

Date _____

HEED goal area	HEED goals assessment score	Change from assessment 1 to assessment 2
Increasing fruits and vegetables		
Decreasing fats		
Increasing dairy and dairy alternatives		
Increasing whole grains		
Balancing calories		
Total score		

HEED Pyramid Assessment

Date _____

HEED pyramid group	HEED pyramid assessment score	Change from assessment 1 to assessment 2
Bread group		
Fruit and vegetable group		
Dairy group		
Meat group		
Fats		
Sweets		

Assessment 3: Session 20

HEED Goals Assessment

Date _____

HEED goal area	HEED goals assessment score	Change from assessment 2 to assessment 3
Increasing fruits and vegetables		
Decreasing fats		
Increasing dairy and dairy alternatives		
Increasing whole grains		
Balancing calories		
Total score		

HEED Pyramid Assessment

Date _____

HEED pyramid group	HEED pyramid assessment score	Change from assessment 2 to assessment 3
Bread group		
Fruit and vegetable group		
Dairy group		
Meat group		
Fats		
Sweets		

APPENDIX B

Daily Food Log

Date: ____________________

My short-term healthy eating goals: ____

____

____

Meal	Food	Amount eaten	Food group (bread, fruits and vegetables, dairy, meat, fats, sweets)	Number of food group servings	Calories (optional)
Break-fast					
Lunch					

(continued)

(continued)

Meal	Food	Amount eaten	Food group (bread, fruits and vegetables, dairy, meat, fats, sweets)	Number of food group servings	Calories (optional)
Dinner					
Snacks					

HEED pyramid food group		Recommended servings per day	My goal servings per day	My servings today ○ = 1 serving
Bread group	*Total*	_____	_____	○○○○○○○○○○○○○
	Whole-grain	(at least 3)	_____	○○○○○○
Fruit and vegetable group	*Total*	_____	_____	○○○○○○○○○○○○
Dairy and dairy alternatives group	*Total*	_____	_____	○○○○○
	Low-fat or fat-free		_____	○○○○○
Meat and meat alternatives group	*Total*	_____	_____	○○○○○
	Lean meat, poultry, fish, legumes, nuts, and soy		_____	○○○○○

Unsaturated fats and oils (list here)

_____

Saturated fats and trans fats (list here)

_____

Sweets (list here)

_____

I attained my short-term healthy eating goals today (circle one): Yes   No

Comments _____

_____

Tips for Achieving Your HEED Goals

This page and the following four pages can be photocopied and placed in a visible place (e.g., on the refrigerator door). Don't feel you have to try all these suggestions—do one or two ideas from the sheet that matches your goals.

Increasing Fruits and Vegetables

1. Begin your day with a breakfast that includes two or more fruit servings.
2. Add dried fruits to cereal, pretzels, and nuts for a quick and easy snack.
3. In a hurry? Buy precut, ready-to-serve fruits and vegetables.
4. Choose fruit for dessert or add a piece of fruit to your favorite dessert.
5. Try a new, or unfamiliar, fruit and vegetable each week.
6. Keep a bowl of cut-up fruit or vegetables on the top shelf of your refrigerator.
7. Take advantage of local farmers' markets for fresh seasonal fruits and vegetables.
8. Use applesauce or prune puree in place of the fat when baking.
9. Add chopped apples, raisins, or blueberries to your favorite low-fat bread, cookie,* or muffin mix.
10. When stir-frying vegetables, decrease the amount of meat by one third and increase the amount of vegetables by one third.
11. Try eating a large salad with at least one meal per day.
12. Increase portion sizes of vegetables by choosing larger pieces or doubling up on servings.
13. Add extra vegetables to your sandwiches, soups, sauces, and casseroles.
14. Reach for a can of vegetable juice instead of a soft drink for a midday pick-me-up.
15. Put color on your plate by including red, purple, orange, yellow, and dark green vegetables every day.

*Same as *biscuit* in some countries.

Decreasing Fats

1. Use low-fat milk or fat-free half-and-half instead of cream in coffee.

2. Try mustard, low-fat dressing, salsa, or low-fat yogurt instead of mayonnaise, sour cream, or butter on sandwiches and baked potatoes.

3. Choose low-fat cooking methods such as steaming, grilling, boiling, and baking.

4. Control the amount of toppings on your foods by asking for salad dressings and sauces to be served on the side.

5. Try butter substitutes instead of butter or margarine on pasta, potatoes, rice, and popcorn.

6. Limit menu items described as fried, creamed, scalloped, or au gratin or that are served with hollandaise.

7. When selecting meats, look for the words *loin* or *round,* such as sir*loin,* top *round,* and *round* steak.

8. Cook poultry with its skin to retain moisture. Then discard the skin before serving.

9. Use low-fat cheese or low-fat, calcium-fortified soy cheese instead of higher-fat cheeses.

10. At buffets, fill your plate with fresh leafy green salads, fresh fruits, and vegetables.

11. Use two egg whites for one whole egg in recipes.

12. Use lean 98% fat-free ground* turkey or lean ground* sirloin instead of ground* beef.

13. At restaurants, ask that vegetables and other side dishes be cooked without added butter or margarine.

14. Take a lunch to work so that you are not tempted to eat out. People tend to eat more fat when eating out.

15. Limit fast food visits or order the child-sized meal for greater portion control.

*Also referred to as *minced* in some countries.

From *Healthy Eating Every Day,* by Ruth Ann Carpenter and Carrie E. Finley, 2005, Champaign, IL: Human Kinetics. Organizations and agencies may not photocopy any material for professional or organizational use or distribution.

Increasing Dairy
and Dairy Alternatives

1. Top your fruit salad with low-fat yogurt and almond slices.

2. Try a refreshing Berry Blue Smoothie to start your morning: Mix 1 cup (240 ml) of nonfat or low-fat milk, a handful of fresh or frozen blueberries, and a dash of honey. Add some ice cubes to make it extra thick.

3. Choose low-fat string cheese or calcium-fortified soy cheese for a quick, high-calcium snack.

4. Try different types of fat-free or low-fat yogurt until you find the variety you like best.

5. Look for new milk products such as fruit-flavored milk, yogurt smoothies, or low-fat cheese cubes in your local supermarket.

6. Add Parmesan or grated Romano cheese to salads and pasta dishes.

7. Try to drink a glass of nonfat or low-fat milk with at least one meal per day.

8. Drink calcium-fortified orange juice with your breakfast.

9. For a fun family project make your own low-fat cheese and vegetable pizzas.

10. Drink the nonfat or low-fat milk that you add to your favorite breakfast cereal.

11. Include cooked, dried beans as a calcium boost to your meal.

12. Stir-fry calcium-fortified tofu and vegetables for a fast and easy snack or meal.

13. Look for calcium-fortified breakfast cereals in the supermarket.

14. Add a cup (240 ml) of nonfat or low-fat milk to a can of condensed cream of celery, mushroom, broccoli, chicken, or tomato soup. Heat and serve.

15. Take calcium-citrate tablets to supplement your diet if you know that it is lacking in dairy foods or calcium.

Increasing Whole Grains

1. Sprinkle a couple of spoonfuls of 100% bran cereal on your favorite breakfast cereal.

2. Use whole-wheat flour for up to one third of the white flour called for in recipes.

3. Buy 100% whole-grain breads with three or more grams of fiber per slice.

4. Add barley or brown rice to soups that have a broth base.

5. Choose a mix of brown or wild rice instead of all white rice.

6. Add flavor and texture by choosing whole-grain breads made with added nuts, seeds, and dried fruits.

7. For a change of pace, choose whole-grain pita pockets.

8. Try cereals that are whole grain and high in fiber such as shredded wheat, oat bran, granola, and muesli.

9. Choose oatmeal for breakfast a few times a week.

10. Experiment with new and unusual grains such as amaranth, quinoa (keen-wah), bulgur, kashi, or spelt.

11. On the labels of grain foods (bread, cereal, pasta, and the like) make sure the first ingredient has "whole" or "stone-ground" in it.

12. Make low-fat bran muffins for an easy-to-carry, fiber-packed snack.

13. Snack on air-popped or low-fat microwave popcorn.

14. Give whole-grain pasta a try or mix it with regular pasta in equal portions.

15. Make whole-wheat pancakes and top with fresh fruit.

From *Healthy Eating Every Day,* by Ruth Ann Carpenter and Carrie E. Finley, 2005, Champaign, IL: Human Kinetics. Organizations and agencies may not photocopy any material for professional or organizational use or distribution.

Balancing Calories

1. Only eat when you are truly hungry.

2. Stop eating when you are comfortably full, not when you are overfull!

3. Watch portion sizes of *all* foods.

4. Include your high-calorie favorite foods but eat them less often and in smaller portions.

5. Eat slowly! You can eat a lot of calories in a short amount of time if you are not mindful.

6. Limit your intake of added sugars and alcohol.

7. Pick up an active hobby such as dancing, gardening, officiating youth sports games, playing a sport, or volunteering as a guide at the zoo.

8. Rent or buy an exercise video for bad weather days.

9. Look for ways to burn more calories during the day. Take the stairs, park farther away, and go for brief, brisk walks.

10. Wear a step counter (pedometer) to monitor your movement throughout the day.

11. Take active vacations or holidays such as hiking or trekking, biking, canoeing, and camping.

12. Clean your home and lawn with vigor! Pick up the pace while you vacuum, scrub, sweep, make beds, dust, rake, and shovel.

13. Walk or ride a bike to do some of your local errands.

14. Record everything you eat and drink and your physical activity each day.

15. Avoid all-you-can-eat buffets, especially if you find that you have trouble controlling your portions in such settings.

From *Healthy Eating Every Day,* by Ruth Ann Carpenter and Carrie E. Finley, 2005, Champaign, IL: Human Kinetics. Organizations and agencies may not photocopy any material for professional or organizational use or distribution.

HEED Goals Assessment

Increasing Fruits and Vegetables

How often do you . . .

▌ Eat at least one serving of citrus fruit* (e.g., orange, grapefruit, lemon, or lime) or citrus fruit juice† per day?

0 points	1 point	3 points	5 points	Score
Rarely or never	1-3 times per week	4-5 times per week	6-7 times per week	_____

▌ Eat at least one serving* of dark green, deep orange, yellow, or red fruits or vegetables per day?

0 points	1 point	3 points	5 points	Score
Rarely or never	1-3 times per week	4-5 times per week	6-7 times per week	_____

▌ Choose fruits or vegetables as a snack instead of choosing a typical snack food?

0 points	1 point	3 points	5 points	Score
Rarely or never	1-3 times per week	4-5 times per week	6 or more times per week	_____

▌ Try new ways to prepare, eat, or order fruits and vegetables?

0 points	1 point	3 points	5 points	Score
Rarely or never	1 time per month	2 times per month	3 or more times per month	_____

▌ Select fruits or vegetables as side dishes when eating out?

0 points	1 point	3 points	5 points	Score
Rarely or never	1-2 times per month	3-4 times per month	5 or more times per month	_____

*1 serving = 1 medium-sized piece of fruit; 1/2 cup (85 g) chopped raw, cooked, frozen, or canned fruit or vegetables; 1/4 cup (35 g) dried fruit; 1 cup (55 g) leafy raw vegetables

†1 serving = 3/4 cup (6 oz; 180 ml) fruit or vegetable juice

Increasing Fruits and Vegetables Score (total) _____ out of 25

Decreasing Fats

Do you . . .

▧ Use butter, margarine, or oils when cooking or as spreads?

0 points	3 points	5 points	Score
Usually choose butter, stick (hard) margarine, shortening, animal fat, or lard	Usually choose whipped or light (reduced-fat) butter or regular tub (soft) margarine	Usually choose liquid margarine, vegetable oils, or reduced-fat tub (soft) margarine	_____

▧ Use salad dressing or mayonnaise?

0 points	3 points	5 points	Score
Usually choose regular option	Usually choose low-fat option	Usually choose nonfat option	_____

▧ Eat beef, pork, lamb, or veal? (Give yourself five points if you rarely or never eat beef, pork, lamb, or veal.)

0 points	3 points	5 points	Score
Rarely choose lean cuts or lean ground* beef, and rarely remove excess fat before cooking or eating	Sometimes choose lean or extra-lean cuts or lean ground* beef, and sometimes remove excess fat before cooking or eating	Usually choose lean or extra-lean cuts or lean ground* beef, and usually remove excess fat before cooking or eating	_____

▧ Eat turkey, chicken, or other poultry? (Give yourself five points if you rarely or never eat any type of poultry.)

0 points	3 points	5 points	Score
Usually choose fried poultry cooked with skin (and you eat the skin) or regular ground* poultry	Sometimes choose baked, broiled, or grilled poultry; poultry cooked with skin (but you don't eat the skin) or lean ground* poultry	Usually choose baked, broiled, or grilled poultry; poultry cooked and eaten without skin; or lean ground* poultry	_____

▧ Eat fish, shellfish, or seafood?

0 points	3 points	5 points	Score
Usually choose fried fish	Sometimes choose fried fish	Usually choose baked, broiled, or grilled fish	_____

▧ Eat cheese?

0 points	3 points	5 points	Score
Usually choose regular option	Sometimes choose low-fat option	Usually choose nonfat or low-fat option	_____

Choose the light or low-fat version of foods and sauces when available?

0 points	1 point	3 points	5 points	Score
Rarely or never	1-3 times per week	4-5 times per week	6 or more times per week	_____

Use the following preparation methods?

0 points	3 points	5 points	Score
Usually fry or saute	Sometimes bake, broil, steam, or grill	Usually bake, broil, steam, or grill	_____

Decreasing Fat Score (total) _____out of 40

Increasing Dairy and Dairy Alternatives

How often do you . . .

Drink milk or soy milk?

0 points	1 point	3 points	5 points	Score
Rarely or never	1-6 times per week	1 time per day (7 times per week)	2 or more times per day	_____

Eat yogurt or soy yogurt?

0 points	1 point	3 points	5 points	Score
Rarely or never	1-6 times per week	1 time per day (7 times per week)	2 or more times per day	_____

Eat natural or processed cheese or soy cheese (cubed, sliced, or shredded)?

0 points	1 point	3 points	5 points	Score
Rarely or never	1-3 times per week	4-5 times per week	6 or more times per week	_____

Eat soft cheeses such as cottage cheese or ricotta cheese?

0 points	1 point	3 points	5 points	Score
Rarely or never	1-3 times per week	4-5 times per week	6 or more times per week	_____

Eat calcium-fortified foods or drinks such as orange juice, cereal, tofu, bread, or pasta?

0 points	1 point	3 points	5 points	Score
Rarely or never	1-3 times per week	4-5 times per week	6 or more times per week	_____

Increasing Dairy and Dairy Alternatives Score (total) _____out of 25

Increasing Whole Grains

How often do you . . .

Eat at least three servings* of whole-grain foods per day?

0 points	1 point	3 points	5 points	Score
Rarely or never	1-3 times per week	4-5 times per week	6-7 times per week	_____

Eat whole-grain ready-to-eat or hot cereal?

0 points	1 point	3 points	5 points	Score
Rarely or never	1-3 times per week	4-5 times per week	6 or more times per week	_____

Eat whole-wheat bread or rolls for sandwiches, toast, or at meals?

0 points	1 point	3 points	5 points	Score
Rarely or never	1-3 times per week	4-5 times per week	6 or more times per week	_____

Eat whole-grain pasta, brown rice, or other whole-grain side dishes?

0 points	1 point	3 points	5 points	Score
Rarely or never	1-3 times per week	4-5 times per week	6 or more times per week	_____

Eat popcorn or whole-grain snacks?

0 points	1 point	3 points	5 points	Score
Rarely or never	1-3 times per week	4-5 times per week	6 or more times per week	_____

Eat whole-grain foods that you haven't tried before?

0 points	1 point	3 points	5 points	Score
Rarely or never	1 time per month	2 times per month	3 or more times per month	_____

*1 serving = 1 slice of bread; one 6-inch tortilla; 1 ounce (30 g, or about 1 cup) ready-to-eat cereal; 1/2 cup cooked cereal (120 g), pasta (70 g), rice (80 g), or sweet corn (80 g)

Increasing Whole Grains Score (total) _____ out of 30

Balancing Calories

How often do you . . .

Read food labels to see how many calories are in foods?

0 points	1 point	3 points	5 points	Score
Rarely or never	1-3 times per week	4-5 times per week	6 or more times per week	_____

Track your daily caloric intake by writing down what you eat or by keeping track in your head?

0 points	1 point	3 points	5 points	Score
Rarely or never	1-3 days per week	4-5 days per week	6-7 days per week	_____

Adjust how much you eat based on the amount of physical activity or exercise you get each day?

0 points	1 point	3 points	5 points	Score
Rarely or never	1-3 times per week	4-5 times per week	6 or more times per week	_____

Make an effort to limit your portion sizes?

0 points	1 point	3 points	5 points	Score
Rarely or never	1-3 times per week	4-5 times per week	6 or more times per week	_____

Choose low-calorie foods and beverages when available?

0 points	1 point	3 points	5 points	Score
Rarely or never	1-3 times per week	4-5 times per week	6 or more times per week	_____

Eat when you are not hungry?

0 points	1 point	3 points	5 points	Score
6 or more times per week	4-5 times per weel	1-3 times per week	Rarely or never	_____

Balancing Calories Score (total) _____ out of 30

Healthy Eating Every Day Score

Now that you've evaluated the different parts of your diet, transfer your total scores for each goal area to the space provided. Add all of your scores to get your grand total.

Increasing fruits and vegetables _____ out of 25

Decreasing fats _____ out of 40

Increasing dairy and dairy alternatives _____ out of 25

Increasing whole grains _____ out of 30

Balancing calories _____ out of 30

Grand total _____ out of 150

REFERENCES

1. Carpenter, R.A., Finley, C., and Barlow, C.E. 2004. Pilot-test of a behavioral skill building intervention to improve total diet quality. *Journal of Nutrition Education and Behavior* 36: 20-26.

2. Appel, L.J., Moore, T.J., Obarzanek, E., Vollmer, W.M., Svetkey, L.P., Sacks, F.M., Bray, G.A., Vogt, T.M., Cutler, J.A., Windhauser, M.M., Lin, P.H., Karanja, N., Simons-Morton, D., McCullough, M., Swain, J., Steele, P., Evans, M.A., Miller, E.R., and Harsha, D.W., for the DASH Collaborative Research Group. 1997. A clinical trial of the effects of dietary patterns on blood pressure. *The New England Journal of Medicine* 336: 1117-24.

3. Sacks, F.M., Svetkey, L.P., Vollmer, W.M., Appel, L.J., Bray, G.A., Harsha, D., Obarzanek, E., Conlin, P.R., Miller, E.R., Simons-Morton, D.G., Karanja, N., and Lin, P.H., for the DASH Collaborative Research Group. 2001. Effects on blood pressure of reduced dietary sodium and the Dietary Approaches to Stop Hypertention (DASH) diet. *The New England Journal of Medicine* 344: 3-10.

4. Obarzanek, E., Sacks, F.M., Voomer, W.W., Bray, G.A., Miller, E.R., Lin, P.H., Karanja, N.M., Most-Windhauser, M.M., Moore, T.J., Swain, J.F., Bales, C.W., and Proschan, M.A. 2001. Effects on blood lipids of a blood-pressure-lowering diet: The Dietary Approaches to Stop Hypertension (DASH) trial. *American Journal of Clinical Nutrition* 74: 80-89.

5. U.S. Department of Agriculture, Agricultural Research Service. 2000. Pyramid servings intakes by U.S. children and adults: 1994-96, 1998 [Online]. ARS Community Nutrition Research Group Web site. Available: www.barc.usda.gov/bhnrc/cnrg/ [April 5, 2004].

6. Social Survey Division. Office of National Statistics. 2003. The National Diet and Nutrition Survey: Adults aged 19-64, energy, protein, carbohydrate, fat, and alcohol intake [Online]. Available: www.statistics.gov.uk/downloads/theme_health/NDNS_V2.pdf [June 29, 2004].

7. Young, L.R., and Nestle, M. 2002. The contribution of expanding portion sizes to the U.S. obesity epidemic. *American Journal of Public Health* 92: 246-49.

8. Centers for Disease Control and Prevention. 2004. Trends in intake of energy and macronutrients—United States 1971-2000. *Morbidity and Mortality Weekly Report* 53(4): 80-82.

9. Cleveland, L.E., Moshfegh, A.J., Albertson, A.M., and Goldman, J.D. 2000. Dietary intake of whole grains. *Journal of the American College of Nutrition* 19(3): 331S-38S.

10. Quatomoni, P.A., Copenhafer, D.L., D'Agostino, R.B., and Millen, B.E. 2002. Dietary patterns predict the development of overweight in women: The Framingham Nutrition Studies. *Journal of the American Dietetic Association* 102(9): 1240-46.

11. Schnoll, R., and Zimmerman, B.J. 2001. Self-regulation training enhances dietary self-efficacy and dietary fiber consumption. *The Journal of the American Dietetic Association* 101: 1006-11.

12. Kant, A.K., and Graubard, B.I. 2004. Eating out in America, 1987-2000: Trends and nutritional correlates. *Preventive Medicine* 38: 243-49.

13. French, S.A., Story, M., Nevmark-Sztainer, D., Fulkerson, J.A., and Hannan, P. 2001. Fast food restaurant use among adolescents: Associations with nutrient intake, food choices and behavioral and psychosocial variables. *International Journal of Obesity* 25: 1823-33.

14. Urbszat, D., Herman, C.P., and J. Polivy. 2002. Eat, drink, and be merry, for tomorrow we diet: Effects of anticipated deprivation on food intake in restrained and unrestrained eaters. *Journal of Abnormal Psychology* 111(2): 396-401.

15. Economic Research Service, USDA. Briefing room: Food CPI, prices, and expenditures. Table 1 Food and alcoholic beverages: Total expenditures [Online]. Available: www.ers.usda.gov/Briefing/CPIFoodAndExpenditures/ [April 5, 2004].

16. Putnam, J., Allshouse, J., and Kantor, L.S. 2003. U.S. per capita food supply trends: More calories, refined carbohydrates, and fats. *ERS FoodReview* 25(3): 2-15.

17. McAuley E., Jerome, G.J., Elavsky, S., Marquez, D.X., and Ramsey, S.N. 2003. Predicting long-term maintenance of physical activity in older adults. *Preventive Medicine* 37: 110-18.

18. Liu, S., Willett, W.C., Manson, J.E., Hu, F.B., Rosner, B., and Colditz, G. 2003. Relation between changes in intakes of dietary fiber and grain products and changes in weight and developments of obesity among middle-aged women. *American Journal of Clinical Nutrition* 78: 920-27.

19. Kant, A.K., Schutzkin, A., Graubard, B.I., and Schairer, C. 2000. A prospective study of diet quality and mortality in women. *Journal of the American Medical Association* 283(16): 2109-15.

20. Rozin, P., Kobnick, K., Pete, E., Fischler, C., and Shields, C. 2003. The ecology of eating: Smaller portions in France than in the United States help explain the French Paradox. *Psychological Science* 14: 450-54.

21. Gillman, M.W., Rifas-Shiman, S.L., Frazier, A.L., Rockett, H.R., Camargo, C.A., Field, A.E., Berkey, C.S., and Colditz, G.A. 2000. Family dinner and diet quality among older children and adolescents. *Archives of Family Medicine* 9(3): 235-40.

22. U.S. Department of Agriculture, Agricultural Research Service. 1997. Data tables: Results from USDA's 1994-96 continuing survey of food intake by individuals and 1994-96 diet and health knowledge survey, table set 10. On: 1994-96 Continuing Survey of Food Intakes by Individuals and 1994-96 Diet and Health Knowledge Survey. CD-ROM, NTIS Accession Number PB98-500457.

23. Blair, S.N., Kampert, J.B., Kohl, H.W., Barlow, C.E., Mareca, C.A., Paffenbarger, R.S., and Gibbons, L.W. 1996. Influences of cardiorespiratory fitness and other precursors on cardiovascular disease and all-cause mortality in men and women. *Journal of the American Medical Association* 276(3): 205-10.

24. Kampert, J., Blair, S.N., and Barlow, C.E. 1999. How much does cardiorespiratory fitness increase longevity? *Medicine and Science in Sports and Exercise* 31: S138.

25. Huang, Y., Macera, C.A., Blair, S.N., Brill, P.A., Kohl, H.W., and Kronenfeld, J.J. 1998. Physical fitness, physical activity, and functional limitation in adults aged 40 and older. *Medicine and Science in Sports and Exercise* 30(9): 1430-35.

26. Bassett, D.R., Schneider, P.L., and Huntington, G.E. 2004. Physical activity in an Old Order Amish community. *Medicine and Science in Sports and Exercise* 3(1): 79-85.

27. Dunn, A.L., Marcus, B.H., Kampert, J.B., Garcia, M.E., Kohl, H.W., and Blair, S.N. 1999. Comparison of lifestyle and structured interventions to increase physical activity and cardiorespiratory fitness: A randomized trial. *Journal of the American Medical Association* 281: 327-34.

28. Sevick, M.A., Dunn, A.L., Morrow, M.S., Marcus, B.H., Chen, G.J., and Blair, S.N. 2000. Cost-effectiveness of lifestyle and structured exercise interventions in sedentary adults: Results of Project *ACTIVE*. *American Journal of Preventive Medicine* 19: 1-8.

29. Flegal, K.M., Carroll, M.D., Ogden, C.L., and Johnson, C.L. 2002. Prevalence and trends in obesity among US adults, 1999-2000. *Journal of the American Medical Association* 288(14): 1723-27.

30. Australia Bureau of Statistics. 2003. Australian Social Trends: Health risk factors among adults [Online]. Available: www.abs.gov.au/Ausstats/abs@.nsf/0/4D5FA8D86976832BCA256D39001BC345?Open [June 29, 2004].

31. Sturm, R. 2002. The effects of obesity, smoking, and drinking on medical problems and costs. Obesity outranks both smoking and drinking in its deleterious effects on health and health costs. *Health Affairs* 21(2): 245-53.

32. NIH/NHLBI. 1998. Clinical guidelines on the identification, evaluation and treatment of overweight and obesity in adults. The evidence report. National Institutes of Health. *Obesity Research* 6(suppl 2): 51S-209S.

33. Wei, M., Kampert, J.B., Barlow, C.E., Nichaman, M.Z., Gibbons, L.W., Paffenbarger, R.S., Jr., and Blair, S.N. 1999. Relationship between low cardiorespiratory fitness and mortality in normal-weight, overweight, and obese men. *Journal of the American Medical Association* 282(16): 1547-53.

34. Matthiessen, J., Fagt, S., Biltoft-Jensen, A., Beck, A.M., and Ovesen, L. 2003. Size makes a difference. *Public Health Nutrition* 6(1): 65-72.

35. Klem, M.L., Wing, R.R., McGuire, M.T., Seagle, H.M., and Hill, J.O. 1997. A descriptive study of individuals successful at long-term maintenance of substantial weight loss. *American Journal of Clinical Nutrition* 66: 239-46.

36. Epel, E., Lapidus, R., McEwen, B., and Brownell, K. 2001. Stress may add bite to appetite in women: A laboratory study of stress-induced cortisol and eating behavior. *Psychoneuroendocrinology* 26(1): 37-49.

37. Oliver, G., Wardle, J., and Gibson, E.L. 2000. Stress and food choice: A laboratory study. *Psychosomatic Medicine* 62: 853-65.

38. Neumark-Sztainer, D., Hannan, P.J., Story, M., Croll, J., and Perry, C. 2003. Family meal patterns: Association with sociodemographic characteristics and improved dietary intake among adolescents. *Journal of the American Dietetic Association* 103: 317-22.

39. Nielsen, S.J., and Popkin, B.M. 2003. Patterns and trends in food portion sizes, 1977-1998. *Journal of the American Medical Association* 289: 450-53.

40. Pimental, D., and Pimental, M. 2003. World population, food, natural resources, and survival. *World Futures* 59: 145-67.

41. Pimental, D., and Pimental, M. 1996. *Food, energy, and society.* Niwot, CO: Colorado University Press.

42. Pimental, D. In press. Livestock production and energy use. In: Cleveland, C.J., ed. *Encyclopedia of energy.*

43. Haddad, E.H., and Tanzman, J.S. 2003. What do vegetarians in the United States eat? *American Journal of Clinical Nutrition* 78(suppl): 626S-32S.

44. McGuire, M.T., Wing, R.R., Klem, M.L., and Hill, J.O. 1999. Behavioral strategies of individuals who have maintained long-term weight losses. *Obesity Research* 7(4): 334-41.

INDEX

Note: The italicized *f* and *t* following page numbers refers to figures and tables, respectively.

ABOUT THE AUTHORS

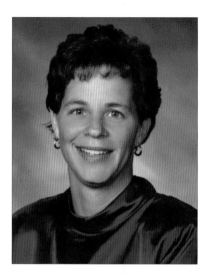

Ruth Ann Carpenter, MS, RD, LD, is the director of the center for research dissemination at The Cooper Institute in Dallas, Texas. She is a registered dietitian with a master's degree in applied nutrition and additional coursework in exercise science.

Carpenter has directed The Cooper Institute's nutrition research for 15 years and was the codeveloper and a group facilitator for the Lifestyle Nutrition Study, which served as the basis for *Healthy Eating Every Day*.

She has coauthored five books, including *Active Living Every Day*, and developed educational programs for clients such as the American Heart Association, Kellogg's, Tropicana, PowerBar, Jenny Craig, Novartis, and Roche. She serves as secretary for the American Dietetic Association's (ADA) weight management dietetic practice group and is a member of the ADA's sports, cardiovascular, and wellness dietetic practice group.

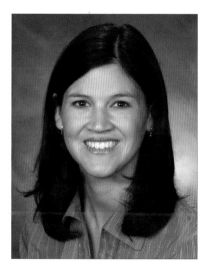

Carrie E. Finley, MS, is a project manager in the center for data management at The Cooper Institute. She codeveloped the curriculum for the Lifestyle Nutrition Study and was a cofacilitator in the program, which provided the framework for *Healthy Eating Every Day*.

Finley manages the nutritional epidemiology project at The Cooper Institute with the goal of studying the associations among dietary intake, fitness, and health outcomes. With a master's degree in epidemiology and a bachelor's degree in nutritional sciences, she is skilled in understanding the impact of dietary habits on health and behaviors.

Finley lives in Dallas, Texas, with her husband, Jeff, and son, Travis.

Continue to improve your quality of life with these additional resources!

 ## Healthy Eating Every Day—It's More Than a Book

The *Healthy Eating Every Day (HEED)* book is one component of an exciting program. In addition to using this book, you can also choose to enroll in HEED Online, in which you'll be able to electronically track your progress and get additional information, assistance, and links to helpful resources. HEED Online is not a replacement of the book, it works in tandem with the book to provide you with a fun, interesting, and helpful interactive experience to promote healthy eating.

You can also take HEED in a classroom setting. For more information, or to enroll, visit www.ActiveLiving.info or call 1-800-747-4457.

HEED Online · ISBN 0-7360-5565-7

 ## Active Living Every Day

Active Living Every Day is a unique behavior change course designed to help adults become and stay physically active. The course uses a variety of behavior change strategies to help you fit physical activity into your daily life in realistic ways that you can maintain over time. The *Active Living Every Day* participant package has everything you need to get and stay moving. It includes the following:

- Access to and support from the Active Living Partners Web site
- *Active Living Every Day* book (also available separately)
- Online study guide
- Online journal

You can take *Active Living Every Day* in a classroom setting or online via the Internet. To locate an Active Living Community Center in your area or to purchase the *Active Living Every Day* participant package, visit www.ActiveLiving.info or call 1-800-747-4457.

Active Living Every Day participant package · ISBN 0-7360-4433-7

Healthy Eating Every Day and *Active Living Every Day* are courses offered by Active Living Partners, a comprehensive behavior change initiative developed by Human Kinetics and The Cooper Institute.

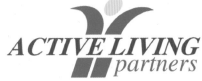

Building Healthy Lifestyles Together
P.O. Box 5076 · Champaign, IL 61825-5076
www.ActiveLiving.info

To place your order, U.S. customers call
(800) 747-4457
Canada: (800) 465-7301 · **Australia:** (08) 8277 1555
New Zealand: (09) 448 1207 · **Europe:** +44 (0) 113 255 5665

2335